Counseling Clients Near the End of Life

James L. Werth, Jr., PhD, is professor of psychology and director of the Doctor of Psychology (PsyD) program in counseling psychology at Radford University, Radford, Virginia. He served as the associate editor for end-of-life issues for the journal *Death Studies* for many years. Dr. Werth has published/edited/coedited approximately 100 articles/book chapters, several special journal issues, and several books, primarily focused on end-of-life issues, ethics, suicide, and HIV disease. As the American Psychological Association's 1999–2000 HIV Congressional Policy Fellow, he worked in the office of Senator Ron Wyden (D-OR) on HIV, aging, and end-of-life issues. Dr. Werth is a licensed psychologist who provides pro bono counseling. He serves on the Board of Directors for the Virginia Rural Health Association, is the rural health coordinator for the Virginia Psychological Association, and is a member of the American Psychological Association's Committee on Disability Issues in Psychology.

Counseling Clients Near the End of Life

A Practical Guide for Mental Health Professionals

James L. Werth, Jr., PhD
Editor

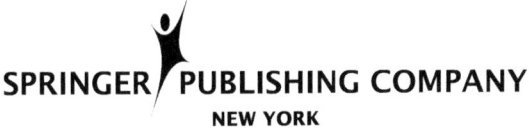

SPRINGER PUBLISHING COMPANY
NEW YORK

Copyright © 2013 Springer Publishing Company, LLC

All rights reserved.

No part of this publication may be reproduced, stored in a retrieval system, or transmitted in any form or by any means, electronic, mechanical, photocopying, recording, or otherwise, without the prior permission of Springer Publishing Company, LLC, or authorization through payment of the appropriate fees to the Copyright Clearance Center, Inc., 222 Rosewood Drive, Danvers, MA 01923, 978-750-8400, fax 978-646-8600, info@copyright.com or on the Web at www.copyright.com.

Springer Publishing Company, LLC
11 West 42nd Street
New York, NY 10036
www.springerpub.com

Acquisitions Editor: Sheri W. Sussman
Production Editor: Michael O'Connor
Composition: Techset

ISBN: 978-0-8261-0849-4
E-book ISBN: 978-0-8261-0850-0

Printed by LSI

The author and the publisher of this Work have made every effort to use sources believed to be reliable to provide information that is accurate and compatible with the standards generally accepted at the time of publication. The author and publisher shall not be liable for any special, consequential, or exemplary damages resulting, in whole or in part, from the readers' use of, or reliance on, the information contained in this book. The publisher has no responsibility for the persistence or accuracy of URLs for external or third-party Internet websites referred to in this publication and does not guarantee that any content on such websites is, or will remain, accurate or appropriate.

Library of Congress Cataloging-in-Publication Data
Counseling clients near the end of life : a practical guide for mental health professionals / edited by James L. Werth Jr.
  p. ; cm.
  Includes bibliographical references and index.
  ISBN 978-0-8261-0849-4 — ISBN 978-0-8261-0850-0
  I. Werth, James L.
  [DNLM: 1. Counseling—methods. 2. Terminal Care—psychology. 3. Caregivers—psychology. 4. Palliative Care—psychology. 5. Patients—psychology. WB 310]
  616.02'9—dc23

2012034010

Special discounts on bulk quantities of our books are available to corporations, professional associations, pharmaceutical companies, health care organizations, and other qualifying groups.

If you are interested in a custom book, including chapters from more than one of our titles, we can provide that service as well.

For details, please contact:
Special Sales Department, Springer Publishing Company, LLC
11 West 42nd Street, 15th Floor, New York, NY 10036-8002s
Phone: 877-687-7476 or 212-431-4370; Fax: 212-941-7842
Email: sales@springerpub.com

I dedicate this book to my parents and my wife, all of whom have had serious health scares during the time that this book was in development.

The fierce commitment that my mother and father demonstrated as each of them received surprise diagnoses of cancer, and each ended up in the hospital, demonstrated the true meaning of partnership. My sister's willingness to drop everything and help out during these trying times was remarkable.

Finally, when my wife, Theresa, woke up exhibiting the symptoms of a stroke while at a conference many hours from home, I wasn't sure what to expect when I arrived at the hospital. Fortunately, she had been rushed to a stroke center, received excellent care, and has fully recovered. Her two sons, Paul and Campbell, and I are very happy that she is back to her spirited self.

The strength and resilience of all of these important people in my life have continued to amaze and inspire me.

Contents

Contributors xi
Preface xiii
Acknowledgments xv

I END-OF-LIFE SERVICE PROVISION

1. Ethical Challenges When Counseling Clients Nearing the End of Life 3
   Louis A. Gamino and Michael B. Bevins
   Hospital-Based Palliative Care 4
   Outpatient End-of-Life Counseling 11
   Conclusion 22

2. Diversity Considerations With Clients Who Are Near the End of Life 25
   Jung Kwak and Elise P. Collet
   Older Adults 26
   Racial, Ethnic, and Cultural Diversity 32
   Relationships Among Race, Ethnicity, and Culture and End-of-Life Experiences 33
   Spiritual and Religious Diversity 37
   Case Examples 42
   Conclusion 44

3. Advance Directives: Planning for the End of Life 53
   Rebecca S. Allen, Morgan K. Eichorst, and JoAnn Oliver
   Characteristics Predicting Completion of Advance Directives 54
   Shared Decision Making 58
   Capacity Evaluations and Undue Influence 61
   Advance Directives and Mental Health 62
   Advance Directives in Long-Term Care 64
   Advance Directives in Acute Care or During the Last Weeks or Days of Life 65
   Interventions to Increase Advance Care Planning and Execution of Advance Directives 66
   Conclusion 68

4. Health Care Teams Working With People Near the End of Life   75
   Kimberly Hiroto and Julia Kasl-Godley
   Health Care Teams Defined   76
   Teams Providing Palliative Care   78
   Team Organization   80
   Factors Affecting Team Organization   81
   Methods to Enhance Team Organization   90
   Conclusion   94

II   WORKING WITH CLIENTS WHO ARE DYING

5. Counseling Clients Who Are Near the End of Life   101
   James L. Werth, Jr.
   Preliminary Considerations   102
   Client's Capacity to Make Decisions   103
   Bio-Psycho-Socio-Spiritual Issues to Review   104
   Social Support System Issues to Review   113
   Systemic and Environmental Issues to be Reviewed   116
   Use of Assessment Instruments With Dying Clients   117
   Conclusion   118

6. Lifespan Considerations for People Who Are Near the End of Life   121
   Illene Noppe Cupit, Deirdre M. Radosevich, and Gail E. Trimberger
   Children and Adolescents and the End of Life   123
   Emerging Adults, Young Adults, and the End of Life   126
   Middle Age and Dying   130
   Older Adults and the End of Life   132
   Conclusion   138

7. Mental Health Symptom Management for Clients Who Are Near the End of Life   141
   Jackson P. Rainer and Johnathan C. Martin
   Decision Making and Diagnosis   143
   Anxiety Disorders   145
   Mood Disorders   147
   Delirium   150
   Personality Disorders   152
   Trauma   154
   Substance Abuse and Dependence   157
   Role of the Clinician: Easing the End of Life   160

8. Cognitive Impairment Near the End of Life   165
   Mary M. Lewis and Jessica M. Moeller
   Types of Cognitive Impairment   166
   Counseling Interventions Appropriate for Individuals With Cognitive Impairment Near the End of Life   171

Critical Issues for Individuals With Cognitive Impairment
Near the End of Life   173
Conclusion   179

III ASSISTING LOVED ONES

9. Counseling the Caregivers of Clients Who Are Near
the End of Life   185
Deborah P. Waldrop and Abbie M. Kirkendall

   Caregiving and the Context for Care Near the End of Life   186
   Experience of Caregiving at Life's End   187
   Conclusion   198

10. Complicated Grief and the End of Life: Risk Factors and Treatment
Considerations   205
Robert A. Neimeyer and Laurie A. Burke

    Features of Complicated Grief   206
    Risk Factors for Complicated Grief   207
    Available Treatments for Bereaved Individuals   216
    Conclusion   224

Index   229

Contributors

Rebecca S. Allen is a professor of psychology at the University of Alabama in Tuscaloosa, Alabama.

Michael B. Bevins is a palliative care physician at the Scott & White Clinic in Temple, Texas.

Laurie A. Burke is a graduate student in the Department of Psychology at the University of Memphis in Memphis, Tennessee.

Elise P. Collet is a graduate student in the Department of Social Work at the University of Wisconsin–Milwaukee in Milwaukee, Wisconsin.

Illene Noppe Cupit is a professor of Human Development and Women's Studies at the University of Wisconsin–Green Bay in Green Bay, Wisconsin.

Morgan K. Eichorst is a graduate student in the Department of Psychology at the University of Alabama in Tuscaloosa, Alabama.

Louis A. Gamino is a psychologist at the Scott & White Clinic in Temple, Texas.

Kimberly Hiroto is a psychologist at the VA Palo Alto Health Care System in Palo Alto, California.

Julia Kasl-Godley is a psychologist at the VA Palo Alto Health Care System in Palo Alto, California.

Abbie M. Kirkendall is an assistant professor of social work at the University of Las Vegas in Las Vegas, Nevada.

Jung Kwak is an assistant professor of social work at the University of Wisconsin–Milwaukee in Milwaukee, Wisconsin.

Mary M. Lewis is a faculty member at Columbus State Community College in Columbus, Ohio, and a psychologist with Senior Life Consultants in Dublin, Ohio.

Johnathan C. Martin is a graduate student in the Department of Psychology at Georgia Southern University in Statesboro, Georgia.

Jessica M. Moeller is a psychologist at the Louis Stokes Cleveland VA Medical Center in Cleveland, Ohio.

Robert A. Neimeyer is a professor of psychology at the University of Memphis in Memphis, Tennessee.

JoAnn Oliver is an assistant professor of nursing at the University of Alabama in Tuscaloosa, Alabama.

Deirdre M. Radosevich is an assistant professor of human development at the University of Wisconsin–Green Bay in Green Bay, Wisconsin.

Jackson P. Rainer is a professor of psychology at Valdosta State University in Valdosta, Georgia.

Gail E. Trimberger is a lecturer in social work at the University of Wisconsin–Green Bay in Green Bay, Wisconsin.

Deborah P. Waldrop is an associate professor of social work at the University of Buffalo in Buffalo, New York.

James L. Werth, Jr. is a professor of psychology at Radford University in Radford, Virginia.

Preface

In a review of the counseling literature, I found very few articles focused on end-of-life issues, and the majority of those that could be placed in this content area were related to aspects such as grief and loss as opposed to providing counseling to persons who were dying and their loved ones (Werth & Crow, 2009). This is remarkable because the American Counseling Association (ACA, 2005) amended its ethics code to specifically include a standard on counseling terminally ill persons (A.9) and referred to this standard within the very important confidentiality section (see B.2.a). The ACA is alone among the large national mental health associations in discussing end-of-life issues in its ethics code, but members of other professions have books aimed directly at them that discuss how they can work with clients who are dying and their loved ones. Similarly, there are dozens of books on working with people after their loved ones have died but there are few resources that address pre-death issues. Thus, this book is designed to fill this gap.

Professional counselors want and need resource material that is practical, evidence-based, and accessible. This book takes these requirements into account by having chapters written by mental health professionals who have experience providing counseling services and, therefore, who can speak from experience, while also basing the information on the empirical literature. The chapters include reader-friendly aspects such as "clinical pearls," which are brief take-home points that have specific, direct relevance to practice and can be put to use by the reader immediately but would not necessarily be obvious to the novice counselor. In addition to these pithy take-home messages, each chapter incorporates at least two cases from the authors' experience to highlight the issues that are raised in the chapter.

The content of the book is based on my own and my colleagues' experience providing counseling to people who are facing end-of-life issues and material appearing in the literature documenting what frontline mental health service providers need to know in order to provide counseling to persons who are dying and their loved ones.

The first section of the book is focused on foundational information that is important for service providers across all types of end-of-life situations.

Louis Gamino and Michael Bevins review ethical challenges and offer a model for addressing these dilemmas. Next, Jung Kwak and Elise Collet provide an overview of diversity considerations and focus on ethnicity/race, older age, and religion/spirituality. In the third chapter, Rebecca Allen, Morgan Eichorst, and JoAnn Oliver review advance directives and how they can be used to assist dying individuals and their loved ones. The final chapter in this first section is on working with teams when providing services to individuals who are dying and their loved ones, and Kimberly Hiroto and Julia Kasl-Godley provide practical tips on how to use teams to their fullest.

The second section of the book focuses on working with clients who are dying. In Chapter 5, I offer a primer of sorts that sets the stage for the more specialized chapters that follow, using a comprehensive framework developed by a Working Group of the American Psychological Association. Then, Illene Noppe Cupit, Deirdre Radosevich, and Gail Trimberger review lifespan considerations and provide information regarding special issues faced by people who are dying at various ages from the very young to the very old. The next chapter focuses on mental health issues, with Jackson Rainer and Johnathan Martin reviewing a number of conditions such as depression and anxiety. The last chapter in this section is by Mary Lewis and Jessica Moeller and they examine the pressing issue of cognitive impairment.

The final two chapters address how to assist loved ones before and after death. Deborah Waldrop and Abbie Kirkendall discuss how to help caregivers when a loved one is dying. Finally, Robert Neimeyer and Laurie Burke provide guidance on helping people who are experiencing complicated grief after the person has died.

I hope that readers will find these chapters useful regardless of whether they are working with their first client who is dying or have been doing this type of work for many years. I know that, as the book's editor, I found myself making my own notes in the margins for things I needed to keep in mind.

REFERENCES

American Counseling Association. (2005). *ACA code of ethics*. Alexandria, VA: Author.

Werth, J. L., Jr., & Crow, L. (2009). End-of-life care: An overview for professional counselors. *Journal of Counseling and Development, 87*, 194–202.

Acknowledgments

As with any big project, there are many people to thank and acknowledge related to this book. Most importantly, I and all the authors thank the people who are dying and their loved ones who give us the privilege of knowing and working with them.

I appreciate all the authors sharing their wisdom and experience with me and everyone reading the book.

Finally, I also appreciate Sheri W. Sussman, the executive editor at Springer Publishing Company, who was patient beyond belief as issues in my own life led to the completion date getting pushed back (see the Dedication). I appreciate my colleagues and students for understanding when I had to be away from teaching and supervising in the midst of these crises.

I

End-of-Life Service Provision

1

Ethical Challenges When Counseling Clients Nearing the End of Life

LOUIS A. GAMINO AND MICHAEL B. BEVINS

"Begin with the end in mind" is a common admonition to goal-oriented individuals who set out on an endeavor attempting to achieve a specific outcome. While all health care, including psychotherapy, is designed to accomplish some salutary purpose, "beginning with the end in mind" has particular significance when treating or counseling clients nearing the end of their lives. The proximity of death as a physical endpoint serves, temporally and existentially, as an organizing principle for the clinician's work with the client and may, in effect, be the "chief complaint." Facilely handling the rigors of end-of-life counseling requires *death competence* on the part of the provider—specialized skill in tolerating and managing clients' problems related to dying, death, and bereavement (Gamino & Ritter, 2009).

Both hospital-based palliative care and end-of-life counseling in outpatient settings generate a host of ethical challenges and dilemmas to consider: ensuring autonomy, assessing capacity for decision making, honoring advance directives, respecting cultural diversity, keeping confidentiality, grappling with medical futility, maintaining boundaries, and including families in the scope of care. Such challenges are not intermittent events but part and parcel of everyday clinical practice. Therefore, conscientious professionals must remain constantly vigilant regarding ethical dilemmas that may arise and remember that "... good counseling practice requires sound ethical practice" (Gamino & Ritter, 2009, p. xviii).

Through the vehicle of case studies, the authors explore and delineate some of the most common ethical challenges that occur when counseling clients nearing the end of life. In the first section, the focus is on hospital-based palliative care where end-of-life counseling involves issues such as how to maximize patient autonomy when deciding whether to stop curative treatment. In the second section, the focus shifts to outpatient settings where end-of-life counseling can strain the boundaries typically enforced in psychotherapy and pose novel challenges to client confidentiality, including *after* death. The authors present a coherent decision-making model to guide clinicians in maintaining ethical integrity when counseling clients under such emotionally charged circumstances.

HOSPITAL-BASED PALLIATIVE CARE

Palliative care is specialized medical care for people with serious illness. Although palliative care is not limited to patients near the end of life or to those foregoing curative treatment, palliative care teams are often called to assist in the care of dying patients and their families. Palliative care is generally delivered by a team, which typically consists of a physician, social worker, and chaplain. This interdisciplinary approach is meant to holistically address patients' physical, emotional, and spiritual needs. Care is typically extended to patients' families as well. In the hospital, clinicians often find patients at a time of crisis or transition in their illness journey. At the same time, patients do not usually stay in the hospital for more than several days, compressing the time available to provide counseling for end-of-life issues. Yet, valuable and meaningful counseling can be performed in this short interval, often precipitating a variety of ethical and legal concerns for clinicians.

CASE 1:

"Ruth" was a 59-year-old woman who drove a school bus until about 18 months ago when she was diagnosed with amyotrophic lateral sclerosis (ALS or "Lou Gehrig's disease")—a neuromuscular disorder that causes progressive weakness, eventually robbing the afflicted of the ability to swallow and breathe. Ruth had been admitted to the hospital four times in the past 6 months for infections and altered mental status caused by retention of carbon dioxide in the blood, which is a consequence of weakness in the breathing muscles. She was confined to bed and unable to speak or swallow on her own. She received artificial feeding through a gastrostomy (stomach) tube, and she required noninvasive assistance breathing by wearing a tight fitting "positive air pressure" mask 24 hours a day. She could, however, still write.

In conversation with multiple physicians, Ruth had consistently expressed her preference not to receive cardiopulmonary resuscitation (CPR) or invasive mechanical ventilation (intubation). However, Ruth's husband had indicated that he would not honor these wishes and instead do whatever he could to keep her alive as long as possible. Ruth and her husband had two adult children living out of state.

During her final hospital admission, the palliative care team was called to assist in Ruth's care. The team met Ruth alone in her hospital room. She was visibly fatigued, but able to write with some effort and communicated that she was in no discomfort. When the team asked about her preferences regarding CPR and intubation, she reiterated her desire not to have either. Ruth knew she was nearing the end of her life and wanted to "go peaceful." She was aware of her husband's intention to request CPR and intubation, but was unsure if he would be allowed to do so against her wishes.

As stated in the American Counseling Association's (2005) *Code of Ethics*, counselors should work to "enable clients to exercise the highest degree of self-determination possible" (p. 5). Preserving and promoting a patient's self-determination is a fundamental aspect of ethical care at end of life. The ethical norm of respecting a patient's right to self-determination is often expressed as the principle of autonomy (Beauchamp & Childress, 2008). Simply put, when a person enters into a therapeutic relationship, she retains the right to determine what is done to her and for her. Respect for autonomy is fundamental to Western biomedical ethics, and is the basis for practices such as obtaining informed consent for treatment and employing advance directives. Accelerated by the exposure of unscrupulous human subjects research and by prominent court cases asserting patients' rights to determine their own medical care, the discipline of bioethics emerged, in the United States at least, as a way to extend and protect the rights of patients (Jonsen, 1998; Rothman, 1991). It is worth bearing in mind, however, that people from non-Western cultures may value autonomy differently; for example, placing more value on the individual's role within the family or community than on the individual's personal interests.

Though the principle of respecting patients' self-determination is now firmly entrenched in medical ethics and in American case law, the reality of making treatment decisions for individual patients can get complicated. Not every patient is able or willing to make her own decisions. Often the first step is to determine if the patient has the *capacity* to make the decision being considered. Capacity is not the same as *competence*, the latter being a legal determination that can only be made by a judge or jury. Capacity has four components: understanding the medical condition; understanding the proposed treatment or test including the risks, benefits, and alternatives; using reason to make a decision; and communicating his or her decision (Miller & Marin, 2000; Sessums, Zembrzuska, & Jackson, 2011).

Capacity is task relative. In other words, a patient may have the ability to make some decisions but not others. For example, a patient might be able to decide if she wants medicine to ease her pain, but may not be able to make the more complex decision about whether to undergo surgery to repair an aortic aneurysm. Because a person's capacity can change over time, it is important to evaluate capacity at the time each decision is to be made. Furthermore, one should avoid making generalized or blanket statements about a patient's lack of decision-making capacity, which risk limiting the person's ability to make whatever decisions she can. Capacity assessments can take a long time, and often require extended interviews. Unfortunately, the contemporary health care system often does not allow sufficient time to fully evaluate a patient's capacity to make decisions. A clinician in a counseling role who has come to know the patient well can often provide valuable information to the medical team regarding capacity.

CASE 1: (*continued*)

In Ruth's case, it was clear that she had the capacity to decide to forego CPR and invasive ventilation. She had consistently expressed this preference over time. In her case, the assessment was tedious because she was very fatigued and could communicate only by writing. Her husband was not present during the assessment. The team first validated Ruth's decision and then explored with her what could happen when she is no longer able to communicate her wishes. Such a situation was foreseeable and inevitable. If her husband were present to demand CPR and intubation, it is likely that Ruth's wishes would be overruled. Of note, the palliative care physician felt Ruth would likely die within days. This short time frame, coupled with Ruth's husband's infrequent presence at the hospital, made it unlikely the team would be able to adequately address his concerns regarding Ruth's decision. It was imperative, therefore, to empower Ruth to take steps to protect herself from receiving undesired medical interventions.

Any patient can defer end-of-life medical decision making to someone else. Some patients prefer that their family members make decisions on their behalf, including people from non-Western cultures. If a patient lacks the capacity to make a decision, most states have laws directing decision-making authority to pass down a hierarchy of individuals related to the patient. The list may vary by jurisdiction, but usually consists of the patient's spouse (but usually not unmarried life partners), adult children, parents, siblings, and available next of kin. In Ruth's case, when she became incapacitated, her husband would have the legal right to make decisions on her behalf. If he were unavailable or unwilling to do so, authority would have passed to the majority of her adult children.

There were several options for helping protect Ruth's self-determination. It is important to know what tools are available in the practitioner's jurisdiction. For example, many states now have POLST (Physician Orders for Life-Sustaining Treatment) or a similar program. Such programs allow physicians to write orders for end-of-life care based on the patient's wishes. These orders can accompany the patient to different health care facilities and so carry authority at home, in the hospital, or at a nursing facility without having to be reissued.

In Ruth's jurisdiction, such a program did not exist. Instead, two other legally recognized tools were available from the category of advance directives: directive to physicians and medical power of attorney (MPOA). Basically, with a directive to physicians, the patient states what treatments she does or does not want if diagnosed with a terminal illness. Unfortunately, many clinicians find such directives unhelpful, and they are often overruled by a proxy decision maker (Silveira, Kim, & Langa, 2010). An MPOA can be useful because it allows the patient to appoint a person of her choosing to make decisions on her behalf.

CASE 1: (continued)

Given that Ruth's husband had expressed an unwillingness to follow her wishes, we discussed an MPOA appointing someone else to make the decisions, effectively removing decision-making authority from her husband. Ruth wanted her daughter to decide stating, "She agrees with me." Further complicating matters, Ruth insisted that no one tell her husband of the MPOA. Within a few days of completing her MPOA, Ruth died peacefully one night in the hospital while her husband was at home. Staff notified her daughter by phone when Ruth was close to death, and her daughter asked that Ruth be allowed to die according to her wishes, without CPR or intubation.

Ruth's case demonstrates both the importance of and the difficulties involved in protecting a patient's self-determination. Ruth's request to forego CPR and intubation was difficult for her husband to accept and, ideally, the palliative care team would have helped him address his concerns. The first priority, however, was to protect Ruth's self-determination. Also, it is notable that Ruth's decision was easily accepted by her medical team. In fact, it was the recommendation of Ruth's physicians that she not have CPR or intubation as these interventions would have provided minimal benefit and considerable burden. Jones and Holden (2004) explained how medical providers are less likely to question a patient's capacity for decision making when the patient's preferences correspond with the providers' views. So, providing palliative care is not always so easy, especially when patients or their families request interventions against the advice and judgment of the medical team.

CASE 2:

"Mattie" was an 81-year-old African American woman who came to the hospital because of weakness and shortness of breath. Previously, she had been living alone in a rural community and performing independently all of her activities of daily living (ADLs). She was involved in her local church and often cooked for large gatherings. Her husband and children had died years before, and her only blood relative was a granddaughter whom Mattie had raised and who still lived nearby.

At the time of her hospital admission, Mattie was diagnosed with aplastic anemia resulting in severe *pancytopenia* (low amounts of blood cells and platelets). No treatment was available to reverse the disorder, and a consulting hematologist recommended that Mattie return home with hospice services. But Mattie declined the recommendation and wanted "everything" done. She required almost daily transfusions of blood and platelets and would have been unable to survive long without them. Because her white blood cell counts were so low leaving her vulnerable to infection, anyone entering her room was required to wear a mask.

Both the consulting hematologist and her primary medical team expressed frustration with Mattie's insistence that "everything" be done. Given that she was frail and prone to bleeding, they thought it would be harmful for her to undergo CPR, but she would not agree to have a "do not resuscitate" (DNR) order. Based on what staff believed were irrational decisions, and based on Mattie's habit of abruptly cutting off conversation without much discussion, her physicians were uncertain whether she fully understood her condition and wondered if she had dementia. The palliative care team was consulted to speak with the granddaughter to "convince her" to take Mattie home with hospice care. Her attending physician even considered calling the hospital ethics committee for advice on whether her treatment should be considered futile and therefore could be discontinued.

After obtaining Mattie's permission, the palliative care team met with the granddaughter, who stated she understood her grandmother's condition was irreversible and terminal despite all available treatments. The granddaughter was willing to care for Mattie at home until she died and agreed that CPR should not be attempted. She also insisted that Mattie was "in her right mind" and should be allowed to make her own decisions. Mattie's granddaughter agreed to speak further with her grandmother about the staff's concerns.

The palliative care team then met with Mattie and her granddaughter together, employing common techniques of effective communication, including open-ended questions such as "What have the doctors told you so far about your condition?" and "What would you say is most important to you at this point in your life?" (Back, Arnold,

& Tulsky 2009). This approach proved to be unwelcome. While maintaining a delightful and warm demeanor, Mattie gave cryptic and unrevealing responses to several open-ended questions before concluding, "Well, thank you for coming by." It was perhaps the politest way the team had ever been ejected from a patient's room!

It seemed as though Mattie was insisting on treatments that her medical team thought inappropriate, and even futile. Ethically and legally, medical personnel are not obligated to provide futile treatments, even if a patient wants them (Jonsen, Siegler, & Winslade, 2010). But it can be difficult to determine when a treatment is futile, and physicians are often reluctant to withhold treatment that an otherwise rational patient requests. Further, there is no single, universally accepted definition of futility. One commonly accepted definition of medical futility is when an intervention will not advance the achievement of a particular goal (Kasman, 2004). Others define futility more broadly, as when an intervention has no reasonable chance of benefiting the patient (Schneiderman, 2011). Additionally, patients and their medical teams sometimes have different goals. Therefore, medical teams may call a treatment futile when it fails to achieve their goals.

When questions of treatment futility arise near the end of life, such as with the continuation of life-sustaining interventions when recovery is impossible, it is important to know statutory law in that jurisdiction. In Mattie's state, a hospital ethics committee can determine that treatment is futile. If so determined, the hospital, along with the patient or her proxy, then has 10 days to arrange transfer to another facility before the treatment can be discontinued by the hospital. Conspicuously, the statute does not contain a definition of futility, so the process is almost always adversarial and protracted. It may also be helpful to involve the facility's ethics committee, legal department, and risk management advisors.

Initiating a futility proceeding with a hospital ethics committee is not the only approach to a patient who wants "everything" done. In such cases, it is imperative to explore what is meant by "everything." Patients are not usually demanding that any and all conceivable interventions be performed. A patient might in fact want everything that will facilitate going home, or being comfortable, or living until a grandchild is born. Furthermore, the patient may be expressing fear of abandonment or of anticipated suffering, or distrust of the medical system. Such thoughts and feelings can only be elicited by engaging the patient in a discussion of what is important to her. Quill, Arnold, and Back (2009) proposed a six-step approach for patients who want "everything," the purpose of which is to partner with the patient in achieving identified goals. A constructive approach must surely begin by trying to elicit the patient's goals and values.

In the case of Mattie, the problem was that she did not want to engage in such a discussion. There is some evidence that her reaction to the medical team may have been culturally based. Research supports the notion that different ethnic or racial groups may approach end-of-life decisions differently. For example, African Americans tend to prefer the use of life support and eschew advance care planning (Kwak & Haley, 2005), while having lower rates of utilizing of hospice services (Washington, Bickel-Swenson, & Stephens, 2008). African Americans may also be more likely to use spirituality to cope with illness and death (True et al., 2005). Specific spiritual beliefs may influence treatment preferences among African Americans, such as a belief that the physician is God's instrument, only God can decide life and death, and divine intervention and miracles do occur (Johnson, Elbert-Avila, & Tulsky, 2005). Indeed, patients who strongly believe in deferring to God's will tend to prefer life-prolonging measures when presented with a poor prognosis (Winter, Dennis, & Parker, 2009).

In Mattie's case, it is also possible that she had previously experienced discrimination and medical mistreatment so that her behavior reflected mistrust of the medical establishment and a mechanism to protect her from unfair treatment (Kwak & Haley, 2005). Generalizations based on culture, race, or other personal characteristics are always tenuous and should be viewed skeptically. Because high-quality and ethical end-of-life care requires a degree of cultural competence, clinicians should always strive to be sensitive to their own and their patients' cultural preferences and biases, while avoiding making assumptions about an individual patient based on culture.

CASE 2: *(continued)*

Mattie had expressed belief that her situation was "in God's hands" and that she wanted "everything" done. Rather than being clear statements of treatment preferences, her statements were interpreted as a starting point for discussion. But after Mattie declined to speak further with the palliative care team, the team did not visit her for the next couple of days but remained in touch with her granddaughter. Unfortunately during this time, Mattie and her granddaughter developed an adversarial relationship with Mattie's attending physician, perceiving him to be condescending and belligerent. The palliative care team then met again with Mattie.

A different approach was taken this time. For one thing, Mattie was dying. The blood and platelet transfusions on which she was dependent were of diminishing effectiveness and she had developed transfusion reactions making additional transfusions risky. Contracting an infection had become a negligible concern so the palliative care team entered Mattie's room without masks and knelt by her bed. No attempt was made to draw her out and elicit her understanding of her condition or her concerns and goals. She had made it clear she did not want to participate in such discussions. Her medical situation was explained and she said she understood. The palliative care physician recommended a change in tactics—treat her symptoms but discontinue transfusions. It was stated clearly that Mattie was near the end of her life, which was regrettable, but CPR would not be performed when she died because it would not help her. Mattie looked at the team and said that sounded alright to her. A plan exclusively for comfort care was ordered. Mattie died peacefully and comfortably several days later with her family at her side.

At first blush, it may not seem like much counseling took place with Mattie. Though she was in the hospital for almost 2 weeks, she never engaged in a traditional counseling session. One of the lessons to be learned from Mattie is the need to tailor practice and techniques to the individual patient. Mattie neither wanted nor needed extensive counseling. It might be assumed that anyone facing death must have myriad existential and spiritual concerns to work out before death or that the dying person must need help to find meaning in dying. Many people do need these things, of course, but not everyone does. It seems what Mattie needed most of all was to remain in control of her life and her death, and to resist being drawn into others' notions of what was right for her. The palliative care team was privileged to play a part in Mattie's dying, but in the end they were just along for the ride.

OUTPATIENT END-OF-LIFE COUNSELING

Clients/families come to end-of-life counseling in outpatient or ambulatory treatment settings via three main avenues: current clients who develop a terminal condition during the course of ongoing psychotherapy/counseling, clients who enter mental health treatment specifically because they have been diagnosed with a terminal illness, and hospice patients who seek counseling during the trajectory of their decline. In the following case study, the patient came to psychological treatment after a diagnosis of terminal cancer.

Consistent with standards established by the American Counseling Association (ACA, 2005), resolving ethical dilemmas requires "... a credible model of decision making that can bear public scrutiny and its application" (p. 3). In what follows, the authors utilize the Five P Model for ethical decision making formulated by Gamino and Ritter (2009). Case analysis emphasizes challenges to confidentiality including postmortem disclosures, boundary maintenance in light of multiple relationships, and the role of transference/counter-transference.

CASE 3:

"Ronnie" was a 50ish White male referred for outpatient psychotherapy because of depression related to a diagnosis of advanced (stage IV) prostate cancer discovered 3 years previously. He had radical prostatectomy (i.e., removal of his prostate gland), but did not qualify for chemotherapy. Following his surgery, he became despondent and distant—trying to separate himself from his family so that it would not be so hard on them when he died.

Ronnie had a checkered past. His natural father was never in the picture and his mother remarried a stepfather who physically abused Ronnie. Furthermore, Ronnie considered himself to be a sex addict, treated women as conquests, and flaunted the notion of fidelity. He married and divorced seven times, the last two times to the same woman. She was the mother of his only natural children—fraternal twins—a boy and a girl, age 12. Following Ronnie's last divorce, his daughter went to live with her mother and became estranged from him. Meanwhile, his son was living with him but, when the common authority conflicts of adolescence arose, the son also went to live with his mother and likewise became estranged.

Initially, the psychotherapy focused on Ronnie's depression over his multiple losses: his health, his sexual potency, his career in the Marines and law enforcement, and his family. Two years after cancer surgery, he had a life-changing religious conversion and came to believe that "God allowed [him] to have the prostate cancer to solve the problem" (i.e., sexual addiction). From that point forward, he made it his life's work to "tell people about the Lord." Eight years after his initial cancer diagnosis, and after 5 years in psychotherapy, Ronnie's cancer recurred aggressively and his oncologist gave him a revised prognosis of "weeks to months." Experimental chemotherapy had little effect on his tumor.

At this point, the nature of the psychotherapy changed from addressing family problems to helping Ronnie prepare for death. Specifically, the clinician prodded him to write letters of love and affirmation to his two children in the event that they did not find a way to reconcile. After months of defensive procrastination, he produced two eloquent, loving letters that conveyed unwavering support and deep affection for his children. The clinician asked for and retained copies of these letters, together with appropriately executed releases of information, allowing the clinician to convey the letters to his children in the future if they had not already received them.

Over time, Ronnie developed a tremendous fondness for the clinician and, in the uninhibited style of those who realize they are approaching death, would often exploit the parting handshake to announce in a loud voice before support staff and even other patients, "I love you, Doc!" The nature and duration of the psychotherapeutic relationship made the patient someone who was "difficult to forget."

Ronnie agreed to videotape one of his psychotherapy visits during which he told a very poignant story of encountering a former nemesis from work after he had been diagnosed with cancer. Even though the bump-in occurred in a retail store, Ronnie barked out the other man's name to get his attention and then proceeded to apologize for his obstinate behavior that was so much to blame for their enmity. The other man accepted his apology and they became good friends from that point.

The clinician was so impressed with this story of reconciliation that he asked Ronnie to "tell his story" at a monthly men's prayer breakfast at the clinician's local church. The patient eagerly accepted, partly as a favor to his beloved doctor but primarily because the invitation afforded him a platform for delivering a message of Christian love. By the time the breakfast could be scheduled, Ronnie was too sick to speak in person. However, he signed a release for the clinician to relate a synopsis of his conversion story and show an edited videotape. The response from the men in attendance was overwhelmingly positive, which Ronnie found very gratifying.

As Ronnie's medical situation deteriorated, hospice care was recommended by the oncologist but he resisted that option as "giving up" and sought the clinician's opinion. When the clinician supported transition to hospice, Ronnie finally agreed and the clinician offered to continue psychotherapy via home visits.

Approximately 1 week later, a family friend notified the clinician that Ronnie was dying. The clinician arrived at the residence just a few minutes after he died. The clinician joined in a bedside prayer led by the hospice chaplain and offered condolences to the patient's mother whom the clinician had met several times in the hospital.

The family asked the clinician to deliver one of three eulogies at the funeral because, "You knew him in a way other people didn't." In the clinician's remarks, Ronnie's status as a psychotherapy patient was revealed and his general character was described but no details of the treatment were disclosed. The family subsequently asked for a written copy of the eulogy.

Ronnie's two children were in attendance at the funeral. The clinician carried in a pocket the two letters from Ronnie to his twins. In the receiving line after the service, the clinician mentioned the letters to the twins who both said they had never received such a letter. Both indicated they would like to have their letter so the clinician conveyed the letters to them on behalf of Ronnie.

Several months later, the clinician received high school graduation announcements from the patient's twins. In response, he wrote two congratulatory, affirmative letters declaring that there was no doubt their father was proud of them on this occasion, and that he loved them despite their differences. The clinician's letters were later acknowledged on standard thank-you cards as if they had been a material gift, and each twin seemed genuinely appreciative.

The Five P Model for ethical decision making (Gamino & Ritter, 2009) provides a conceptual structure for higher order, critical-evaluative reasoning that goes beyond an immediate, intuitive response to a situation based only on the facts and ordinary moral sense to incorporate knowledge of statutory law, practice regulations, codes of conduct, and ethical principles (Kitchener, 1984). The Five P Model takes into account the *person* with a challenging ethical *problem* in a particular contextual *place*, while applying appropriate ethical *principles* in a deliberate decision-making *process*.

Person

Who is this person? Ronnie is a middle-aged White male dying of prostate cancer. Formerly "tough" and controlling in his work and personal habits, he came to prize his Christian beliefs as his primary identity and adopted evangelization as his life purpose. Nonetheless, his family relationships with his ex-wife and two children were fractured to the point of estrangement so that his elderly mother was his chief supporter. He developed a close bond with his treating clinician. His "acceptance" of the dying process was mixed and some degree of denial was present in his pursuit of experimental chemotherapy and resistance to hospice.

Problem

What is the specific ethical challenge to be resolved? Actually, three main ethical problems emerge from the case scenario. First, the problems pertaining to confidentiality are prominent throughout the trajectory of care, and after death. To what extent is Ronnie's family, especially his mother, privy to the details of his treatment or involved in decisions regarding chemotherapy or hospice? What about revealing Ronnie's status as a psychotherapy patient at the prayer breakfast and again at his funeral? Can information from the treatment be revealed to participants at the prayer breakfast, to sympathizers hearing the eulogy, or to the children in the letters from the clinician? Is there any justification for these various disclosures? What are appropriate guidelines regarding postmortem disclosures?

Second, the clinician's behavior raises questions about appropriate boundaries as a consequence of multiple relationships. Besides the formal provider–client relationship, the clinician simultaneously took on two other less formal relationships: a "social" one engendered by the invitation to the prayer breakfast that implied status for the client as a peer/friend; and a "personal" one inherent in accepting an invitation to eulogize the client at his funeral (along with two other work associates of the patient). Do these boundary crossings pose either potential harm to Ronnie or impair the clinician's objectivity/neutrality in discharging the functions of the professional role? Did Ronnie have free choice to decline the speaking invitation without affecting his access to continuing treatment? Did the provider inappropriately take advantage of the therapeutic relationship to "further" a personal (religious) agenda?

Third, transference/counter-transference dynamics, if unacknowledged or misunderstood, can cloud the clinician's ability to exercise sound judgment about Ronnie's case. Is the clinician always acting in the best interest of the client guided by core values of beneficence and fidelity, or is the clinician "acting out" a camouflaged personal agenda of attention-seeking or over-identification with the client? Were transference/counter-transference issues thoroughly addressed in the psychotherapeutic encounter so as to minimize or eliminate such problems?

Place

Initially, the grief counseling took place in a traditional office setting wherein the provider was largely in control and the patient was like a "guest." Stringent confidentiality standards existed to protect the patient's health information and demand characteristics of the office environment reinforced conventional provider–client boundaries.

However, the action in this case shifted at one point from an outpatient office to a community setting (i.e., church fellowship hall) and later to a hospital. These alternate settings strongly influence how the provider protects client confidentiality, maintains boundaries, and manages the interpersonal dynamics of the provider–client relationship. For example, in community settings, it is entirely at the client's discretion whether status as a client of the provider, or any other information about treatment, will be disclosed; the provider follows the client's lead. In hospitals, confidentiality is strictly enforced but, given that the hospital room is the patient's "temporary domicile" and/or the fact that the patient's ability to care for self is compromised, family and guests in attendance often participate in evaluations and receive information directly from hospital staff (cf., Gamino & Ritter, 2009).

Beyond these physical designations of place, the end-of-life period may be considered a metaphorical "place" at the terminus of the lifespan with its own unique rules governing ethical behavior. For example, current palliative care standards identify the *family* as the "unit of care" (National Quality Forum, 2006), so dealing with the family network is essential and that may include routine sharing of information with loved ones. Also, physical contact between provider and client—and between provider and family members—at the end of life may involve physical proximity or touch not otherwise typical. Reconsiderations of such traditional provider–client boundaries when counseling near the end of life are displayed in Table 1.1.

TABLE 1.1
Reconsiderations of Provider–Client Boundaries in End-of-Life Counseling

Typical Office Behavior	Topic	Common Practice in End-of-Life Counseling
No disclosures beyond consultation session without specific written/oral permission.	← Confidentiality →	Discussion of client information with family and loved ones, especially when client's consciousness is compromised.
Handshakes at greeting or parting; perhaps occasional hug; rare contact during Gestalt/psychodrama maneuver.	← Physical Contact →	Sitting/standing close; holding hands; touching limb/shoulder; hugging (patient/family); assisting with physical care.
Selective/strategic self-disclosure that advances "process" discussion of "here-and-now." Emotion *described* but generally *not displayed*.	← Self-Disclosure →	Greater demand to be "in the moment" during the transitional period of dying. More disclosure of personal thoughts, feelings, beliefs (e.g., religious convictions). More permissive approach to display of emotion.
More formal, more "vertical" relationship, with power differential favoring the provider. Friendly, but not friend.	← Relationship Dynamic →	Less formal, more "horizontal" relationship, with more equalized power. More "friend-like" or "honorary family."

Principles

The principles that guide ethical decision making near the end of life include not only the traditional quintet of ethical principles—nonmaleficence, beneficence, autonomy, justice, and fidelity (Kitchener, 1984)—but also federal standards, statutory law, case law, practice regulations, and professional codes of ethics. Each of the three ethical challenges posed by the case example draws on different aspects of these factors in order to resolve the dilemma.

Confidentiality, a cornerstone of health care and end-of-life counseling, is based on the ethical principle of fidelity. A fiduciary relationship between provider and client means telling the truth, proving oneself trustworthy with confidences, exercising loyalty to the client, acting with integrity, taking responsibility, and advocating for the client when necessary and appropriate. Fidelity implies that the provider will act in the best interest of the client (i.e., beneficence) and avoid actions or measures that may harm the client (i.e., nonmaleficence). Fidelity flatly prohibits disclosing client health information or pre-empting the client's prerogative to disclose (or not), barring certain exceptional circumstances such as imminent danger to self or others.

The prospect of postmortem disclosures presents a unique challenge to confidentiality. It is important to remember that a *deceased person's right to confidentiality does not expire at death*. The ACA Code of Ethics (2005) directly addresses this topic, "Counselors protect the confidentiality of deceased clients, consistent with legal requirements and agency or setting policies" (p. 8). Families may request a deceased client's medical record, for example, seeking information about the care or the cause of death. Recognizing that physicians need guidance about how to handle such situations, the American Medical Association (AMA) Council on Ethical and Judicial Affairs (2000) urged that a deceased person's medical record be kept confidential to the greatest extent possible and provided guidelines for a judicious approach to such disclosures. Berg (2001) wrote a detailed assessment of conditions that may justify postmortem disclosure of client information. However, Werth, Burke, and Bardash (2002) warned that the public's trust in the enterprise of psychotherapy as a confidential endeavor may be undermined if patients fear that their personal disclosures may one day be revealed after their deaths. Some major considerations to follow when contemplating postmortem disclosure are summarized in Table 1.2.

The boundary issues embedded in the case example arise in large part from the clinician's decisions to assume some degree of personal relationship with Ronnie and his family beyond the confines of a strictly professional stance. Taking on an additional personal or professional association in addition to the original provider–client dyad is referred to as *multiple relationships*. The Code of Ethics of the Association for Death Education and Counseling (ADEC, 2006) contains a clear provision on why assuming multiple relationships is risky:

> Members refrain from multiple relationships if (1) such relationships could reasonably be expected to impair the objectivity, competence, or effectiveness of the member in performing his/her responsibilities; or if (2) such relationships otherwise risk exploitation or harm to the person(s) with whom the professional relationship exists or formerly existed. (ADEC Code of Ethics, II. General Conduct G)

Maintaining objectivity and impartial judgment toward the client pertains primarily to the principle of fidelity. Avoiding exploitation or harm to the client is the personification of nonmaleficence as an ethical principle.

Instances of *boundary crossings*, such as occurred in the case example with the invitation to speak at the prayer breakfast, involve a deliberate decision by the counselor to cross a customary division or separation of roles in order to achieve something helpful or beneficial to the client that

TABLE 1.2
Major Considerations for Postmortem Disclosure of Client Treatment Information

Autonomy
How can the client's right to self-determination regarding release of personal health information be preserved or extended after death?
- Honoring any statements or directives issued by the client prior to death regarding potential disclosure (or not) of health information after death
- Personal representative or next of kin permitting disclosure (or not) based on what the client would have wanted

Beneficence
Will someone gain or benefit from disclosure?
- Family members seeking information pertinent to their health risks
- Public health authorities seeking to protect the general welfare
- Medical researchers seeking cures or remedies

Nonmaleficence
Will the client, or others, be harmed as a result of disclosure?
- Damaging the reputation of the deceased, or his/her associates
- Respecting the sensitivity of the client's personal health information regarding conflicted or problematic relationships with those who may be privy to disclosure
- Protecting the integrity of counseling as an enterprise and reinforcing public trust in its confidential nature

Justice
What is fair treatment for the client and others regarding disclosure?
- Heirs/beneficiaries seeking compensation after "wrongful death"

Fidelity
How to continue advocating for the client after death?
- Remaining wary of personal gain from disclosure (e.g., fame, fortune) that may undermine the professional obligation of confidentiality
- Resisting interest by unrelated third parties (e.g., biographers, media) seeking to circulate/publicize the client's health information

---

may not occur otherwise (cf., Welfel, 2006). In doing so, the counselor must be very vigilant that personal agendas do not hitchhike on the purported goal of helping the client. This injunction is clearly stated in the ADEC (2006) Code of Ethics, "Members do not use their professional relationships to further their personal, political, religious, or business interests" (ADEC Code of Ethics, II. General Conduct E). Because purity of motive is so rare in boundary crossings, Simon and Williams (1999) suggest providers ask themselves, "Am I making this intervention or taking this action for the benefit of the [client's] treatment or for my own personal benefit?" (p. 1441).

Gottlieb (1993) offered a decision-making tool for professionals contemplating whether to assume a second (or third) association with a client. In considering multiple relationships prospectively, Gottlieb encouraged providers to assess the current relationship with the client along three dimensions: *degree of power* the provider exerts in relation to the client;

duration of relationship, with longer relationships implying more influence; and *clarity of termination*, referring to the likelihood of the provider and client having further professional contact. Then, these same considerations are applied to the contemplated relationship. When the counselor's power and influence are high, the duration of the relationship has been or will be lengthy, and termination is ambiguous, multiple relationships should be avoided.

Giving primacy to client welfare should always be evaluated from the perspective of the client (Gottlieb, 1993). Nowhere is this evaluation trickier than when accounting for the roles of therapeutic transference and countertransference in the counseling dynamic. Katz (2006b) warns providers counseling clients nearing the end of life about striking a delicate balance between maintaining a professional perspective as provider and "being present" in a human manner to share the profound vulnerability of the dying process with a client. Her advice is reminiscent of Karl Menniger's oft-quoted dictum, "When in doubt, be human" (Gutheil & Gabbard, 1998, p. 413). The sacred and mysterious aspects of dying create untold elements of ambiguity for providers traversing such delicate emotional territory. Death competence and accurate self-awareness on the part of providers is so crucial in these circumstances that its importance is difficult to overstate. The ADEC (2006) Code of Ethics contains a key provision regarding such self-knowledge among providers, "The member strives to understand his or her death-related feelings and experiences and the ways in which these may impact his or her thinking and work in the field" (ADEC Code of Ethics, Basic Tenets 2).

Process

Having reviewed the ethical principles most applicable to the dilemmas inherent in the case example as well as some of the key statutory and practice-specific guidelines available, the final step in the Five P Model is the process used in resolving the identified dilemmas related to confidentiality, boundaries, and transference/counter-transference. Ideally, the process respects all significant stakeholders in the dilemmas and allows all pertinent "voices" to be heard when deliberating a decision.

Regarding confidentiality, Ronnie was clearly "in charge" of his health information in the early stages of the case example and permitted his mother to be included in some discussions of his care status. Although this assurance of confidentiality became a bit more ambiguous in the hospital setting when his mother was present at the time of the clinician's visits, it was a relatively simple matter for the clinician to ask for some time alone with Ronnie, or to clarify if he wanted/needed the consultation to be private or "communal." Such an approach kept Ronnie in charge of any disclosures.

The use of the Ronnie's image/voice (via videotape) and basic case information at the prayer breakfast constituted a clear departure from the usual type of information release (e.g., transmission from one health care provider to another). In that instance, the recipients of the information were congregation members of a specific church. When the plan was for Ronnie to present his "story" in person, he retained complete prerogative to share whatever information about himself that he wished. However, once Ronnie was unable to speak in person, the clinician obtained written permission to disclose treatment information at the breakfast. A formal release document notwithstanding, deciding how much to disclose required sensitivity and judgment on the part of the clinician to avoid bringing any harm to Ronnie as a result (e.g., sullied reputation) or unnecessarily conveying any other "protected health information" (Health Insurance Portability and Accountability Act, 1996).

Similarly, the clinician had Ronnie's written permission to convey his affirmation letters to the children—permission he gave knowing full well it was the clinician's belief that the children should receive them. Technically, according to statutory law in the jurisdiction of record (e.g., Texas), only Ronnie's personal representative could authorize disclosure of the letters to the children after his death (Texas Rules of Evidence, 1998; Vernon's Texas Codes Annotated, 1998). Clearly, the clinician preempted this line of authority. By operating according to Ronnie's declared "pre-mortem" intentions that his children receive the letters (see Table 1.2), the clinician could argue that the "spirit of the law" guided the decision because the clinician was carrying out Ronnie's (autonomous) intent (cf. Werth et al., 2002). The clinician acknowledged that delivery of these letters felt like a posthumous "mission accomplished" of therapy work urging Ronnie to seek reconciliation with his children as part of "the four things that matter most" near the end of life (Byock, 2004).

Delivering a eulogy at the funeral de facto revealed Ronnie's status as a psychotherapy patient and included insights into his character acquired through the treatment. Again, understanding Ronnie's wishes regarding postmortem disclosure was a major consideration. The clinician reasoned that Ronnie would be more than happy to reveal to anyone that he was in therapy if he thought it might "help someone else get to heaven." Because the family invited the clinician to give a eulogy, their request implied the prospect of receiving comfort from the provider's remarks. To the extent that Ronnie's family and others would be helped by the clinician's eulogy, the standard of beneficence as a rationale for postmortem disclosure could be invoked. At the same time, guarding against a mere sating of curiosity by others about Ronnie's treatment demanded selectiveness (i.e., fidelity), and avoiding references to family conflicts ensured a minimum of risk to the family's or Ronnie's reputations (i.e., nonmaleficence).

Likewise, when the clinician subsequently received graduation announcements from the patient's children, competing considerations came into play. Above all, protecting confidentiality was still required. Yet ordinary rules of social courtesy call for a response to written invitations. By writing letters of congratulations that reiterated the patient's pride in his children, the provider adopted a type of proxy position by speaking words on behalf of the patient that he could no longer deliver himself. Again, the potential "gain" in helping the children seemed to be the strongest argument for writing while any possible postmortem harm to the patient seemed negligible. In the end, a simple act of human kindness appeared to be the proper response.

In regard to crossing traditional boundaries by inviting Ronnie to speak at the church prayer breakfast, one question was whether this action was therapeutic or exploitative. The invitation could be seen as giving a dying man an otherwise unavailable opportunity to "witness" to fellow Christians about how cancer changed his life in a positive way, thereby affording him a chance to find meaning in his suffering, practice altruism, and generate a positive outcome from a negative life event—all consistent with Ronnie's self-professed evangelical mission. Yet embedded in the invitation was an alteration in the dynamic of the provider–client relationship brought about by introducing a peer association as fellow believers.

This "softening" of the formal boundaries in the context of end-of-life counseling (see Table 1.1) was judged to be less worrisome in light of it being a single event and in consideration of the impending, final termination of the treatment relationship at death (cf., Gottlieb, 1993). The clinician discussed with Ronnie possible "collateral consequences" of presenting at the prayer breakfast, for example, enhanced status for the provider because of recruiting a speaker, displaying a successful example of professional work, and being admired by the client. Ronnie perceived the invitation as an honor and an "obligation" not to the provider, but to his "Higher Power." From Ronnie's perspective, if presenting made his doctor "look good" in the process that was merely well-deserved recognition incidental to the real purpose of witnessing about his faith beliefs. He did not feel exploited but rather grateful for the opportunity.

However at another level, the invitation to the prayer breakfast brought up the issue of counter-transference and the need for self-awareness (Katz, 2006a). Mulling over this invitation beforehand required the clinician to consider the role of several possibilities: over-determined helping (i.e., doing *more* than what was professionally indicated), over-identification with the client (i.e., sharing a faith life), over-involvement with the client (i.e., enacting friendship), or unfilled needs of the provider (i.e., enhancing status in the church community). In the end, the decision was influenced somewhat by the "small town" setting where overlapping relationships tend to be more common and more tolerated (Gripton & Valentich, 2004) and fidelity is maintained by compartmentalizing roles, not relationships (Barnett & Yutrzenka, 1994). In retrospect, the clinician acknowledged that utilizing peer consultation prior to extending this invitation may have been a helpful way to assure "stereoscopic" accuracy regarding several possible interior motivations (cf., Gamino & Ritter, 2009).

The request by Ronnie's family for the provider to deliver a eulogy at the funeral involved counter-transference elements as well. In this case, even though the clinician did not seek out this invitation, it nonetheless tapped into unexpressed interior aspirations to "preach" (even though ministry had not been chosen as a life vocation). Accordingly, the clinician weighed whether accepting was more about meeting the family's apparent need or gratifying a personal desire. Asking what Ronnie would have wanted was a critical consideration and the answer to that question clearly seemed to be affirmative (i.e., he would have readily endorsed the idea as a good one). Thus, accommodating the family's wishes and inferring Ronnie's preferences constituted the primary reasons why the invitation was accepted—to accomplish something beneficial for the family as the "unit of care"—while the clinician's personal aspiration remained an (undisclosed) secondary factor.

CONCLUSION

The case examples detailed in this chapter illustrate some of the key ethical issues that arise in counseling clients nearing the end of life. In hospital settings, autonomy over treatment preferences and end-of-life decision making is paramount. Treating the family as the unit of care in palliative care is important. Delivering clinical care in concert with adherence to legal and ethical considerations can be tricky. In hospice or clinic settings, issues pertaining to confidentiality and boundaries require special attention. In all cases, the counselor must be well aware of the operation of transference and counter-transference forces that may influence the nature and course of the provider–client interaction in salutary or deleterious ways while at all times maintaining client welfare as the highest priority.

REFERENCES

American Counseling Association. (2005). *ACA code of ethics*. Retrieved from http://www.counseling.org

American Medical Association Council on Ethical and Judicial Affairs. (2000). *Confidentiality of health information postmortem* (Rep. No. 5-A-00). Available from the American Medical Association Ethics Standards Group. Chicago, IL: Author.

Association for Death Education and Counseling (ADEC). (2006). *Code of ethics*. Retrieved from http://www.adec.org/about/ethics.cfm

Back, A., Arnold, R., & Tulsky, J. (2009). *Mastering communication with seriously ill patients*. New York: Cambridge University Press.

Barnett, J. E., & Yutrzenka, B. A. (1994). Nonsexual dual relationships in professional practice, with special applications to rural and military communities. *The Independent Practitioner, 14*, 243–248.

Beauchamp, T. L., & Childress, J. F. (2008). *Principles of biomedical ethics* (6th ed.). New York: Oxford University Press.

Berg, J. (2001). Grave secrets: Legal and ethical analysis of postmortem confidentiality. *Connecticut Law Review, 34*, 81–122.

Byock, I. (2004). *The four things that matter most: A book about living*. New York: Simon & Schuster.

Gamino, L. A., & Ritter, R. H., Jr. (2009). *Ethical practice in grief counseling*. New York: Springer Publishing.

Gottlieb, M. C. (1993). Avoiding exploitive dual relationships: A decision-making model. *Psychotherapy, 30*, 41–48.

Gripton, J., & Valentich, M. (2004). Dealing with non-sexual professional–client dual/multiple relationships in rural communities. *Rural Social Work, 9*, 216–225.

Gutheil, T. G., & Gabbard, G. O. (1998). Misuses and misunderstanding of boundary theory in clinical and regulatory settings. *American Journal of Psychiatry, 155*, 409–414.

Health Insurance Portability and Accountability Act of 1996, 45 C.F.R. Parts 164.508-512. Retrieved from www.cms.hhs.gov/HIPAAGenInfo

Johnson, K. S., Elbert-Avila, K. I., & Tulsky, J. A. (2005). The influence of spiritual beliefs and practices on the treatment preferences of African Americans: A review of the literature. *Journal of the American Geriatrics Society, 53*, 711–719.

Jones, R. C., & Holden, T. (2004). A guide to assessing decision-making capacity. *Cleveland Clinic Journal of Medicine, 71*, 971–975.

Jonsen, A. R. (1998). *The birth of bioethics*. New York: Oxford University Press.

Jonsen, A. R., Siegler, M., & Winslade, W. J. (2010). *Clinical ethics: A practical approach to ethical decisions in clinical medicine* (7th ed.). New York: McGraw-Hill.

Kasman, D. L. (2004). When is medical treatment futile? A guide for students, residents, and physicians. *Journal of General Internal Medicine, 19*, 1053–1056.

Katz, R. S. (2006a). The journey inside: Examining countertransference and its implications for practice in end-of-life care. In R. S. Katz, & T. A. Johnson (Eds.), *When professionals weep: Emotional and countertransference responses in end-of-life care* (pp. 269–283). New York: Routledge.

Katz, R. S. (2006b). When our personal selves influence our professional work: An introduction to emotions and countertransference in end-of-life care. In R. S. Katz, & T. A. Johnson (Eds.), *When professionals weep: Emotional and countertransference responses in end-of-life care* (pp. 3–9). New York: Routledge.

Kitchener, K. S. (1984). Intuition, critical evaluation and ethical principles: The foundation for ethical decisions in counseling psychology. *The Counseling Psychologist, 12*, 43–55.

Kwak, J., & Haley, W. E. (2005). Current research findings on end-of-life decision making among racially or ethnically diverse groups. *The Gerontologist, 45*, 634–641.

Miller, S. S., & Marin, D. B. (2000). Assessing capacity. *Emergency Medicine Clinics of North America, 18*, 233–242.

National Quality Forum. (2006). *A national framework and preferred practices for palliative and hospice care quality*. Retrieved from: http://www.qualityforum.org/Publications/2006/12/palliative_hospice_full.aspx

Quill, T. E., Arnold, R., & Back, A. L. (2009). Discussing treatment preferences with patients who want "everything." *Annals of Internal Medicine, 151*, 345–349.

Rothman, D. J. (1991). *Strangers at the bedside*. New York: Basic.

Schneiderman, L. J. (2011). Defining medical futility and improving medical care. *Bioethical Inquiry, 8*, 123–131.

Sessums, L. L., Zembrzuska, H., & Jackson, J. L. (2011). Does this patient have medical decision-making capacity? *The Journal of the American Medical Association, 306*, 420–427.

Silveira, M. J., Kim, S. Y. H., & Langa, K. M. (2010). Advance directives and outcome of surrogate decision making before death. *New England Journal of Medicine, 362*, 1211–1218.

Simon, R. I., & Williams, I. C. (1999). Maintaining treatment boundaries in small communities and rural areas. *Psychiatric Services, 50*, 1440–1446.

Texas Rules of Evidence, Rule 509 (f)(1), Physician–Patient Relationship. (1998).

True, G., Phipps, E. J., Braitman, L. E., Harralson, T., Harris, D., & Tester, W. (2005). Treatment preferences and advance care planning at end of life: The role of ethnicity and spiritual coping in cancer patients. *Annals of Behavioral Medicine, 30*, 174–179.

Vernon's Texas Codes Annotated, Occupations Code §159.005 (a)(5), Consent for Release of Confidential Information. (1998).

Washington, K. T., Bickel-Swenson, D., & Stephens, N. (2008). Barriers to hospice use among African Americans: A systematic review. *Health & Social Work, 33*, 267–274.

Welfel, E. R. (2006). *Ethics in counseling & psychotherapy: Standards, research, & emerging issues* (3rd ed.). Belmont, CA: Thomson Brooks/Cole.

Werth, J. L., Jr., Burke, C., & Bardash, R. J. (2002). Confidentiality in end-of-life and after-death situations. *Ethics & Behavior, 12*, 205–222.

Winter, L., Dennis, M. P., & Parker, B. (2009). Preferences for life-prolonging medical treatments and deference to the will of God. *Journal of Religion and Health, 48*, 418–430.

2

Diversity Considerations With Clients Who Are Near the End of Life

JUNG KWAK AND ELISE P. COLLET

Near the end of life, each person prepares for and faces challenges differently. The uniqueness of each individual's end-of-life experiences is determined by varying illnesses, preferences for types and site of care, and how to communicate and make decisions about end-of-life care, access to care, and outcomes at the end of life. This variety near the end of life stems from a number of factors that include, but are not limited to, the person's physical condition, sociodemographic characteristics, racial/ethnic and cultural backgrounds, and religious and spiritual beliefs.

The major goals for counseling patients and families near the end of life are to recognize this diversity and identify and relieve suffering that is imposed by diseases and treatments on clients within their unique physical, psychosocial, cultural, and religious and/or spiritual contexts. In working to achieve these goals, counselors can assist patients and families in communication and decision making about goals for care and treatments and avoid an unnecessarily prolonged dying process. In addition, they can provide counseling to assess and meet physical, psychosocial, and spiritual needs to promote and support opportunities to achieve a sense of control and completion; communicate with loved ones; and experience a sense of spiritual and existential transcendence (Tilden, Tolle, Drach, & Hickman, 2002). Although variability in the way people cope with their end-of-life challenges is influenced by a myriad of factors, it is especially important for counselors to pay attention to factors such as a person's developmental stage (e.g., older adults), race/ethnicity and associated cultural influences, and religiosity and or spirituality.

Because of marked increases in life expectancy and the survival of more Americans to late life, older adults make up the majority of those dying each year (Lunney, Lynn, & Hogan, 2002). Older adults have special needs that are distinct from younger individuals who are near end of life, and older adults are more likely to be affected by comorbidities of varying severity as well as a greater level of functional impairment and need for care (World Health Orgnization, 2004) that require attention from counselors working in a variety of care settings. Recognizing the important role of race, ethnicity, and associated cultural norms and values on how each client responds to his or her illness and end-of-life challenges is another important area of consideration. Counselors now work with increasingly diverse client populations as the United States has become more multiracial and multiethnic. An individual's racial and ethnic identity and associated culture have a profound influence on how the person perceives and attributes meaning to illness and suffering, communicates needs and concerns, seeks and accesses care, and grieves (Krakauer, Crenner, & Fox, 2002; Kwak, Allen, & Haley, 2011; Kwak & Haley, 2005). In order to provide culturally sensitive care with clients in this multiracial and multiethnic society, it is critical to understand the role of disparities in access and outcomes near the end of life and differences and similarities in beliefs, preferences, and behaviors regarding end-of-life issues among diverse groups of clients and their families. Finally, spirituality/religiosity near the end of life is an important area of great diversity and significance as sources of distress as well as resources in coping with challenges (National Consensus Project for Quality Palliative Care, 2009; Puchalski et al., 2009).

In the following sections of this chapter, we provide a brief overview of three major factors related to the diversity of end-of-life experiences—being an older adult, racial/ethnic and cultural backgrounds, and diverse religious faith and spiritual beliefs. Throughout the chapter, particular emphasis is placed on addressing the implications of diverse characteristics of clients and family systems on physical, psychological, social, cultural, and spiritual/religious dimensions. These aspects are considered distinct but interrelated dimensions that affect the experience of the person near the end of life and are grounded in the bio-psycho–social–spiritual framework articulated by Kaut (2006) and consistent with elements of palliative care identified by practice guidelines from the National Consensus Project for Quality Palliative Care (2009). We pay specific attention to areas that are important to address, including communication, decision making, and coping with psychological and spiritual distress near the end of life.

OLDER ADULTS

In assessing needs and developing appropriate care plans to work with older adults and their families near the end of life, it is important for counselors to consider individual, family, and environmental factors that influence a person's perception of his or her needs for care, preferences for and decisions about care, and psychosocial and spiritual/religious concerns. These factors include an older person's physical needs and trajectories of dying, perception of prognosis, quality of life, mental health needs, and family concerns and support needs.

End-of-Life Trajectories

In 2009, over 70% of the approximately 2.5 million deaths in the United States occurred among older adults aged 65 or over (Kochanek, Xu, Murphy, Miniño, & Kung, 2011). The vast majority of older Americans die after living with a prolonged period of multiple debilitating functional impairments and chronic conditions (Lunney, Lynn, Foley, Lipson, & Guralnik, 2003; Lunney et al., 2002). The leading causes of death among the 1.7 million older adults who died in 2009, for example, were chronic illnesses such as heart disease, cancer, respiratory (lung) disease, and stroke (Kochanek et al., 2011). These illnesses accounted for 59% of all deaths, whereas the fifth leading cause of death, accidents, accounted for only 5% of all deaths among older adults. This is in stark contrast to younger adults, who died more often from accidents than any of the diseases.

Understanding the different trajectories of dying associated with these life-threatening illnesses among older adults is important because of the implications for expected length of survival for a given illness, and the impact on end-of-life decisions, quality of life, family concerns and caregiving burden, and psychosocial and spiritual/religious support needs (Kwak et al., 2011). Glaser and Strauss (1968) proposed that, depending on the type of major illness, individuals may experience different durations (e.g., rapid or slow progression toward death) of clinical and functional changes of varying trajectories (e.g., short-term improvements and relapses, crises, plateaus). According to the dying trajectories theory (Glaser & Strauss, 1968; Lunney et al., 2002), there are four modal trajectories: sudden death, terminal illness, organ failure, and frailty (see Table 2.1).

Some people die suddenly without experiencing any significant change in functional ability (i.e., sudden death). Individuals in the terminal illness category are characterized with a reasonably high functional status that rapidly declines within 6 weeks to 3 months before death, which is typically shown among some types of cancer patients. The organ failure group, those with congestive health failure or chronic obstructive disease, experience gradually decreasing functional ability that is often accompanied by periodic exacerbations of symptoms. The last category is the frailty group in which individuals experience slow decline of functional ability with steadily progressive disability as a result of illnesses such as stroke or dementia. Although there can be substantial variability in the way individuals

TABLE 2.1
Special Considerations for Working With Older Adults and Families

Research among older adults near the end of life suggests that varying trajectories of dying have different implications for need and support for older adults and families. This summary of characteristics of four main trajectories and special areas requiring attention from counselors is based on a review of the literature on this topic.

Trajectories of Dying	Characteristics	Areas of Special Attention in Practice
Sudden death	Sudden death without experiencing any significant change in functional ability	The needs of the bereaved at risk of complicated or prolonged grief.
Terminal illness	A reasonably high functional status that rapidly declines within 6 weeks to 3 months before death, typically shown among some types of cancer patients	The needs for practical caregiving and emotional support for family caregivers especially those providing care at home.
Organ failure	Serious organ system failure related to illnesses (e.g., congestive heart failure or chronic obstructive disease) with gradually decreasing functional ability that is often accompanied by periodic exacerbations of conditions	The changing needs for medical care and impact of a series of acute hospitalizations on client and family's goals and expectations for care and potential decisional conflicts.
Frailty	Slow decline of functional ability with steadily progressive disability as a result of illnesses (e.g., stroke or dementia)	Increasing long-term care needs and subsequent transitions between care settings, especially nursing facilities and hospitals. The need for practical caregiving and emotional support for family caregivers, especially those providing care at home and decision-making support for surrogate decision makers.

experience symptom severity and functional decline across various life-threatening conditions (Gott et al., 2007), the majority of older adults who die of organ system failure or frailty spend the last years of their lives in gradual decline of their health and functioning (Lunney et al., 2002). On the other hand, the terminal dying trajectory, which is a relatively brief but intense period of deterioration leading to death, is experienced by the minority of older adults who die of cancer.

Medical conditions affect the perceptions and experiences of individuals differently because clinical characteristics often change over time and current prognostic criteria for many life-threatening conditions lack precision and accuracy (Kwak et al., 2011). The uncertainty in the progression and gradual functional decline associated with these chronic conditions often limits access to specialized palliative or hospice care, and opportunities for clients to explore and address other important tasks such as psychosocial and spiritual/religious concerns near the end of life. Palliative care, according to the World Health Organization (WHO, 2004), is defined as an approach that improves the quality of life of patients with life-threatening illnesses and their families through early identification, assessment, and treatment of pain, as well as other physical, psychosocial, and spiritual problems. In the United States, hospice is the main source of palliative care and is found to benefit terminally ill patients and their families by providing a holistic care approach in response to their unique physical, emotional, social, and spiritual needs and by providing better pain management and quality of care compared to nursing care only at home or traditional care provided at nursing home or hospitals (Teno et al., 2004).

However, under Medicare or most states' Medicaid programs, which are the major sources of financing for hospice care, hospice services are reimbursed only to the patients with terminal illness with a prognosis of less than 6 months and who forego curative treatments. As a result, the current hospice benefit is suited to patients who experience a more predictable trajectory of disease course, such as those with lung cancer. Many older adults who die of conditions with less certain trajectories of decline, such as organ system failure or frailty, do not use hospice care because physicians are reluctant to identify these patients as dying, in part as a result of the difficulties in accurate prognostication of life expectancy (Christakis & Lamont, 2000; Lunney et al., 2003). Consequently, persons with these chronic conditions near the end of life are likely to perceive their life expectancies to be longer than they in fact are and pursue aggressive treatments with goals and expectations to treat underlying conditions, whereas people dying of illnesses with more predictable courses of progression (e.g., certain types of cancer) may choose palliative or hospice care options.

The trajectory of a given illness and uncertainty regarding progression of the illness not only greatly influence how each client appraises his or her illness and prognosis, but also often leads to shifting goals of care and increased transitions between care settings such as hospitals, skilled nursing facilities, homes, and other types of long-term care settings (Kwak et al., 2011; Mezey, Dubler, Mitty, & Brody, 2002). It is this time of transitions between care settings that often requires careful attention from counselors to help patients and families cope with challenges associated with changing conditions and making difficult decisions.

When counseling patients and families during the time of transition, it is important to recognize that each care setting has its own distinctive philosophies, goals of care, and expectations that may be in conflict with those of other care settings, patients, and families (Mezey et al., 2002). For example, although hospitalization is often appropriate for older adults with certain conditions (e.g., organ failure), hospitalization is not necessarily appropriate for all dying patients. When certain frail older adults are transferred to hospitals with a culture of care shaped by a goal of treating underlying illnesses, which often involves aggressive treatments including surgery and life-sustaining treatments (e.g., cardiopulmonary resuscitation, ventilators), hospitalization can result in adverse outcomes such as sudden death, disruption of care plans, disorientation, and unnecessary financial costs (Engel, Kiely, & Mitchell, 2006). Furthermore, decisions regarding transitions in care settings are often initiated by care providers, especially in nursing homes, and made without sufficient planning by families who make decisions at brief, urgent moments of crisis often brought about by abrupt changes in the patients' condition (Levine, Halper, Peist, & Gould, 2010; Sharma, Freeman, Zhang, & Goodwin, 2009). Such transfers between care settings in the last weeks or days of life often lead to discontinuity of care and have been linked to poor outcomes near the end of life, including an overreliance on aggressive treatment (SUPPORT Principal Investigators, 1995), poor communication of treatment preferences among providers and patients, inadequate management of pain and symptoms (Borum, Lynn, & Zhong, 2000; Intrator, Zinn, & Mor, 2004), and inattention to the spiritual needs of patients and families (Hanson, Danis, & Garrett, 1997). Therefore, it is important to consider the care contexts and settings in assessment of end-of-life challenges faced by clients and families and development of care plans to address the changing needs of the patients and families near the end of life.

Physical, Psychological, Spiritual, and Family Concerns

As the client's underlying illness progresses and the client is faced with poor prognosis and impending death, counselors need to assess and identify psychological, social, family, and spiritual/religious concerns. These forms of distress can interfere with the client's ability to function and cope with the challenges of the dying process and death, and limit the opportunities to have meaningful and quality interactions with family, friends, and care providers (Kaut, 2006). The client's quality of life and ability to deal with important life and death issues is affected by different forms of pain and suffering—physical, emotional, social, spiritual, and existential—and each form of suffering has different implications for practice (Kaut, 2006). Careful assessment is needed regarding physical distress such as physical pain and nonpain symptoms such as nausea, fatigue, and weakness as they affect physical function and overall quality of life. Presence of physical pain and functional impairment also affects decisions people make about their care. Studies have shown that patients are less likely to pursue aggressive treatments when suffering (e.g., pain, poor quality of life) is present (Ebell, Doukas, & Simth, 1991) and when significantly impaired cognitive functioning is expected, because people associated decreased cognitive functioning with decreased quality of life (Allen, Hilgeman, & Allen, 2010).

It is also important to consider psychological domains, including fear of dying, sadness, grief (Block, 2001), and dignity (Steinhauser et al., 2000). Any presence of psychiatric illnesses such as anxiety and depression (Block, 2001), and hopelessness and suicide ideation can increase suffering and even the desire for hastened death among people who are terminally ill (Breitbart et al., 2010) and must be carefully assessed and treated. Similarly, the spiritual/religious dimension of the person is a distinct element that can be affected differently by a person's history, illness, and other dimensions such as biological, psychological, and social aspects (Puchalski et al., 2009). Spirituality and/or religiosity plays an important role in maintaining the well-being of a person near the end of life (Steinhauser et al., 2000; Tarakeshwar et al., 2006) and spiritual distress has been shown to reduce quality of life near the end of life (Tarakeshwar et al., 2006). Therefore, counselors need to assess various components of spirituality and religiosity, such as the person's religious beliefs, religious coping and support, spiritual well-being, spiritual need, and existential concerns, and work to address these areas in collaboration with chaplains or other spiritual care providers with appropriate training and skills.

Another area for assessment and support near the end of life is clients' concerns about family members and their need for support. Family members and other important people in clients' lives contribute significantly to clients' well-being and quality of life by providing extensive practical caregiving support and emotional and spiritual care (Kaut, 2006; Salmon, Kwak, Acquaviva, Brandt, & Egan, 2005). Spouses, life partners, family, and friends carry out many important responsibilities such as personal care, transportation, management of pain and other symptoms, and making important medical decisions for the person who is dying. Families are also central to maintaining and strengthening a sense of connectedness and finding meaning and purpose near the end of life.

Although many family members find their role and experience a meaningful opportunity for growth (Salmon et al., 2005), the substantial demand of caregiving, especially near the end of life, can lead to negative psychological and physical health effects (Dumont et al., 2006; Pickens, O'Reilly, & Sharp, 2010). In their role as surrogate decision makers for critical end-of-life issues, many family members report that they are uncertain about their roles and responsibilities, uninformed about treatment options, and feel unsupported by professionals when making these decisions (Ditto, Hawkins, & Pizarro, 2005; Gessert, Forbes, & Bern-Klug, 2000). These unmet needs can lead to treatment delays, increased stress, and caregiving burden (Breen, Abernethy, Abbott, & Tulsky, 2001; Kramer, Boelk, & Auer, 2006).

Furthermore, the death of a loved one has a profound impact on family members. Although the majority of families are resilient in coping with significant loss and grief (Bonanno & Kaltman, 2001), some family members, especially those who experienced loss of the family member because of a sudden, unexpected death such as an accident or suicide, may grieve for a prolonged period of time with debilitating and sometimes life-threatening symptomatology (i.e., complicated grief; Shear et al., 2011; or prolonged grief disorder; Boelen & Prigerson, 2007).

To effectively support clients and family members, counselors need to assess families' understanding of the illness and its consequences for the client as well as the family; caregiving capacities, needs, and coping strategies to identify any areas of need for education, training, and practical support related to physical care of the client; and family concerns about communication with the dying client and health care providers, decision making, and dealing with spiritual and religious matters (Kwak, Salmon, Acquaviva, Brandt, & Egan, 2007; Salmon et al., 2005). In addition, counselors need to pay particular attention to family members who might be at risk of complicated or prolonged grief and develop grief interventions to address these issues among family members in a manner that is consistent with the cultural and spiritual needs of the family.

Counselors need to approach working with older adults and their families near the end of life with a broad understanding of the diverse factors that contribute to each client's experience of dying and death. These issues include changing illness and environmental contexts that influence perceptions, responses to illnesses, needs, and preferences, and shifting priorities in goals of care of the dying person and his or her family near the end of life.

RACIAL, ETHNIC, AND CULTURAL DIVERSITY

Counselors often work with clients and their families from diverse racial/ ethnic and cultural backgrounds. It is projected that members of ethnic minority groups, including Hispanics of all races, will account for 50% of all Americans by 2050 (U.S. Census Bureau, 2004). A similar trend can be found among older adults. The population of ethnic minority older persons is expected to increase rapidly, from 20% of older Americans in 2010 to 42% by 2050 (U.S. Administration on Aging, 2010). A number of studies examining end-of-life experiences of diverse racial/ethnic groups (see reviews by Kwak & Haley, 2005; Krakauer et al., 2002) document that racial/ethnic and cultural backgrounds significantly influence a person's knowledge of, and access to, care options, as well as perceptions, beliefs, communication, and decision making near the end of life. Moreover, there are known disparities in access to, and outcomes of, care near the end of life experienced by persons of ethnic minority backgrounds. Therefore, it is important for counselors to understand how race, ethnicity, and culture may influence end-of-life experiences in order to develop the understanding, skills, knowledge, and attitudes needed to provide effective counseling and support for diverse groups of clients.

In this section, we highlight some of the major issues related to understanding the relationships among race, ethnicity, culture, and end-of-life experiences; provide a brief review of the current literature on disparities in access and outcomes near the end of life; describe the differences and similarities in end-of-life beliefs, attitudes, and behaviors across major racial and/or ethnic minority groups; and discuss implications for culturally sensitive practice with diverse groups of clients and families.

RELATIONSHIPS AMONG RACE, ETHNICITY, AND CULTURE AND END-OF-LIFE EXPERIENCES

Understanding end-of-life experiences from the perspective of racial and ethnic minority populations is clearly a challenging task because of the lack of consensus in conceptual definition and measurement of these concepts and the complex, interrelated relationships among race, ethnicity, and associated cultural heritage. In the past, race had been defined and considered to be an important biological concept in that the genes that determine race were believed to be linked with the genes that determine health (Centers for Disease Control and Prevention, 1993; Egede, 2006). However, most associations between disease and race have been found to have no biological basis and there is general agreement that race is a socially constructed concept of limited biological significance. Ethnicity is another socially constructed category that is determined by genes, culture, and social class; includes wider categories than race; and, therefore, may be a more useful concept, so it has been commonly used in studies on health disparities (Egede, 2006).

The concept of culture as distinct from, but nevertheless related to, race and ethnicity has been proposed as a better explanation for differences in health behavior and outcomes. According to the U.S. Department of

Health and Human Services Office of Minority Health (1999, p. 8), culture is defined as "integrated patterns of human behavior that include the language, thoughts, communications, actions, customs, beliefs, values, and institutions of racial, ethnic, religious, or social groups." Each culture provides explicit or implicit rules of conduct and a language that includes a set of symbols associated with the group. These rules and language are what we turn to in seeking explanations and answers or meaning for our illness and suffering near the end of life (Rio, 2004).

In most health research, including that done regarding end-of-life issues, culture has been considered a valid explanation for racial and ethnic differences in health outcomes (Egede, 2006). However, more often than not, race or ethnicity has been used as a proxy for culture instead of directly measuring specific cultural traits (e.g., values, beliefs, norms) and, thus, cultural explanations for ethnic or racial differences in attitudes, behaviors, and outcomes in health have been speculated and inferred rather than directly tested (Egede, 2006). Similarly, the majority of studies examining ethnic and racial diversity regarding end-of-life matters do not necessarily distinguish the effects of the sociocultural characteristics (e.g., socioeconomic status, discrimination) of racial and ethnic minorities from cultural perceptions about illness and disease that shape the meanings groups assign to end-of-life issues (Kwak & Haley, 2005). Given these conceptual and methodological limitations about the roles of race, ethnicity, and culture near the end of life, it is important to recognize that racial and ethnic differences near the end of life are attributable not only to cultural differences, but also to social and economic inequalities, language barriers, and other disadvantages affecting racial/ethnic minority groups.

Racial/Ethnic Disparities Near the End of Life

Racial and ethnic disparities in end-of-life care have been documented by an extensive body of literature that includes the findings from the SUPPORT study and the Institute of Medicine report *Unequal Treatment: Confronting Racial and Ethnic Disparities in Health Care* (Payne, 2001; Phillips et al., 1996; Smedly, Stith, & Nelson, 2003). Such disparities, defined as "racial or ethnic differences in the quality of health care that are not due to access-related factors or clinical needs, preferences, and appropriateness of intervention" by the Institute of Medicine (Smedly et al., 2003, p. 3), are reported in the areas of cancer diagnostic tests and treatments, symptom and pain management, and use of palliative and hospice care (Borum et al., 2000; Imperato, Nenner, & Will, 1996; Krakauer et al., 2002; Phillips et al., 1996; Smedly et al., 2003). Reasons for disparities in these areas draw from overall disparities in access to care, socioeconomic status, and inadequate translation and interpreter services. Racial and ethnic groups in general have lower educational levels and lower incomes compared to Whites. With limited knowledge and financial resources, persons from minority groups may lack access to health information about services such as early screening and diagnostic tests for varying illnesses and innovative programs such as palliative and hospice care. Non-English–speaking patients' inability to communicate also contributes to a poorer understanding of their prognosis (Intrator et al., 2004) and to limited communication among physicians, patients, and families (Azoulay et al., 2000).

Therefore, for counselors working with racial/ethnic minority clients, it is particularly important to pay attention to the reality of disparities in access to quality care experienced by many persons of minority backgrounds. Counselors can work to build trust and to identify any potential barriers to timely, quality care that a client may experience near the end of life through a careful and comprehensive assessment of the client's social and economic resources and actively advocate for client's concerns as the client navigates the health care system.

Racial and/or Ethnic Influence on End-of-Life

Many studies report that even when socioeconomic factors are taken into account, racial and ethnic differences in end-of-life care remain. These differences are in part attributed to diverse religious and cultural beliefs and norms guiding communication and decision making about illnesses across cultural groups. Persons from racial/ethnic minority backgrounds may be especially likely to turn to their traditional norms and practices near the end of life because these beliefs and norms can provide them with meaning for their illnesses and guide them in making decisions (Ersek, Kawaga-Singer, Barnes, Blackhall, & Koenig, 1998).

Among the major racial and ethnic groups included in research regarding end-of-life preferences and practices, African Americans are the most frequently studied and found to consistently prefer aggressive treatments more than other racial/ethnic groups (Kwak & Haley, 2005). Compared with other groups, African Americans have also been found to be less likely to prefer or use hospice care (Kwak, Haley, & Chiriboga, 2008; Reese, Ahern, Nair, Schorock, & Warren-Weath, 1999) and they are more likely to prefer to die in hospitals and actually do so (Weitzen, Teno, Fennell, & Mor, 2003).

Suggested explanations for African Americans' preference for and use of aggressive treatments include their religious and spiritual beliefs regarding health and illness and the low level of trust in the U.S. health care system. Culturally, traditional African American spiritual, religious, and cultural values are often in disagreement with hospice philosophy and foregoing curative treatments (Blackhall et al., 1999; Burrs, 1995; Waters, 2001).

Traditionally, African Americans believe in God's omnipotence and miracles, especially regarding medical care decisions, and rely on their religious faith for recovery or cure near the end of life rather than accept terminality (Reese et al., 1999). Another explanation is distrust of the overall medical system resulting from the history of discrimination and mistreatment by the medical and health care community, such as the infamous Tuskegee Syphilis Study, and overall disparities in medical care experienced by African Americans (Ersek et al., 1998; Payne, 2001; Reese et al., 1999; Waters, 2001).

Studies of other racial/ethnic minority groups have also documented less favorable attitudes toward advance directives among Native Americans and East Asians (Johnstone & Kanitsaki, 2009; Murphy et al., 1996). Studies on these groups have offered cultural explanations including cultural aversion to direct communication about serious illnesses and poor prognosis among Chinese and Native Americans (Bowman, 2004; Carrese & Rhodes, 1995), and preferences for group consensus and family as a decision-making unit among various ethnic groups such as Japanese, Korean, Chinese, Hispanic, Native Americans, Lebanese, and Bosnian immigrants (Bito et al., 2007; Blackhall et al., 1995; Gebara & Tashjian, 2006; Searight & Gafford, 2005). These ethnic cultures consider talking about death and dying as a cultural taboo, so direct conversations about issues related to dying and death, and therefore communication and planning in advance, is discouraged. Moreover, because these cultures expect families to be actively involved in the decision-making process, including making final decisions on behalf of the person, completing documents such as living wills to provide specific instructions for end-of-life care may seem impractical and of limited utility.

Studies also document different interpretations and coping approaches among people of various cultures, suggesting that counselors may need to be respectful of a number of explanations for the source or origin of the current illness in clients. Instead of explaining illness based on the biomedical model, some cultures may believe illnesses originate from physical, emotional, or spiritual imbalances, fate, or the will of God (Rio, 2004). For example, Cambodians and Laotians believe that illness is a result of imbalance between yin and yang (Keovilay, Rasbreidge, & Kemp, 2000). Thus, counselors need to recognize culturally bound rules and beliefs about origins of a given illness, appropriateness of open communication about dying and death, locus of control regarding health and illness, and decision-making responsibilities and shared authority (Bito et al., 2007; Johnstone & Kanitsaki, 2009).

In addition to the distinct beliefs and norms across various cultural groups, there are also variations among individuals within the same culture and individuals may identify themselves with more than one culture and may adopt beliefs, traditions, and behaviors of other cultural groups (Rio,

2004). Many studies document that the greater diversity within each cultural group stems from a number of sources such as the person's cultural identity, socioeconomic status, religious beliefs, personal beliefs and experiences, acculturation level, geographic location (e.g., rural vs. urban), level of English proficiency, and knowledge of types and utility of end-of-life care treatments and care options (Kwak & Haley, 2005). For example, research on immigrant populations has shown that those who are more acculturated to the host culture have a more positive perception of, and greater use of, advance directives and direct disclosure of prognosis of an illness to the patient (Kwak & Haley, 2005). Therefore, it is also important for counselors to recognize that a "one size fits all" approach to approaching end-of-life issues with clients and families cannot be successful and they must be careful to avoid stereotyping of clients.

In sum, for counselors working with diverse populations near the end of life, it is important to understand and respect diverse health beliefs and practices, learn about cultural values and norms, build trust, and avoid presuming that the views of persons from the same racial/ethnic background are uniform (Kwak & Haley, 2005). It is also important to recognize disparities and barriers to access to care experiences by persons of minority backgrounds and advocate for timely access to quality end-of-life care on behalf of clients and families. Practitioners can assist patients and families from diverse cultures by exploring and respecting the clients' and families' beliefs and practices about explanations for illnesses and methods of healing, communication about dying and death, and the role of family in decision making and caregiving, while addressing concerns about access to quality care options near the end of life, in a culturally sensitive manner for each client and his or her family support system (see Table 2.2).

SPIRITUAL AND RELIGIOUS DIVERSITY

When working with persons who are dying, it is essential for counselors to consider all aspects of the client and his or her support systems, especially spiritual and or religious world views, because these beliefs can provide a sense of meaning, hope, comfort, and strength (Craigie, 2010). It takes knowledge and sensitivity when addressing religious and spiritual beliefs during a client's dying experience, because each client and support system is likely to have a unique religious/spiritual framework. According to a 2011 Gallup poll, the majority of Americans (76.1%) label themselves as either Protestant Christian or Catholic, while the third most common identification is None/Atheist/Agnostic (15%). The rest of the Americans identify themselves as Mormon (1.9%), Jewish (1.6%), Muslim (0.5%), and believers of other religions (2.4%). In addition, people are increasingly shifting their attitude about what being religious/spiritual may mean to them. A 2008

TABLE 2.2
Special Considerations for Working With Racially/Ethnically Diverse Groups of Clients and Families

A large body of literature documents disparities in the end-of-life experience among racially/ethnically diverse groups of individuals and families because of a number of characteristics, including different cultural values and norms associated with the groups. This table provides a brief summary of major between- and within-group differences in attitudes, communication, and decisions regarding end-of-life care from a review of the literature.

Diversity Across Racial/Ethnic Groups	Areas of Special Attention in Practice
Between-Group Differences	
• Disparities in access to and outcomes of care near the end of life	• At-risk minority clients and families with low social and economic resources • Potential barriers and resources in accessing end-of-life care services • Need for education and counseling to guide in exploring care options and decision making and advocacy in the health care system

• Negative attitudes toward and lower completion of advance directives and lower use of palliative and hospice care	• Need for interpreter and translation services
	• Different value orientations among clients regarding end-of-life care communication and decision making
	  ○ Beliefs that life and death is beyond one's control (i.e., fatalism)
	  ○ Religious and spiritual faith in the role of God or Higher Power of healing and recovery from illness
	  ○ Aversion to direct conversations about death and dying and disclosure of poor prognosis to the dying client
	  ○ Families as basic decision-making unit taking a burden of responsibility to make decisions on behalf of the dying client
	• Distrust of the overall health care system and institutions because of history of mistreatment and abuse and current disparities in access to quality of care and health outcomes
	• Need of family members as decision makers for information and practical support (e.g., interpretation, advocacy)

Within-Group Differences	
• Greater variability within than across racial/ethnic groups regarding attitudes toward disclosure, advance directives, and palliative and hospice care	• Sources of within-group differences including sociodemographic factors (e.g., age, gender, education, income), acculturation level, personal experience with illnesses, religious and spiritual beliefs, and location (e.g., rural vs. urban)

Gallup poll that indicates that the number of those who find religion "very important" has decreased by 20% since 1952, illustrates this. As these data reflect, practitioners need to be informed about the changing spiritual/religious values, beliefs, and norms related to health, illness, and death and dying within the diverse populations with whom they are working.

In this section of the chapter, we briefly clarify definitions of some major concepts related to spirituality/religiosity, review the literature on the role of religion/spirituality in end-of-life decisions such as preferences for life-sustaining treatments and euthanasia, as well as end-of-life care outcomes and promising interventions, and offer practice recommendations.

Conceptual Definitions

To better understand the role of spirituality and religiosity in the end-of-life experiences of patients and families, clarification of definitions of several major concepts is needed. For the purpose of this chapter, religiosity is defined as adherence to philosophical tenets of an organized religious system of faith, belief, and practice that nurture the relationship with a divine being or force (McGrath, 2002). Spirituality is more nebulous; for example, a review of the literature on the relationship between spirituality and health found 92 definitions of spirituality (Unruh, Versnel, & Kerr, 2002). We define spirituality as an individual's attitudes, beliefs, and behaviors that are informed by the guidance of historical tenets, cultural values, social influences, and personal introspection (Kaut, 2006). Religion often refers to the outward form of belief, including rituals, dogmas, creeds, denominational identity, and ecclesiastical structures, and spirituality can be considered the inner feelings and the experience of the immediacy of a Higher Power (Cohen, Thomas, & Williamson, 2008). Spirituality is generally considered a broader concept than religion and within the religious domain, spirituality can be described as a sense of connectedness to a personal God, whereas in the secular domain spirituality is perceived as a search for significance and meaning (Chochinov & Cann, 2005). It is also useful to recognize that both religiousness and spirituality are multidimensional in nature in that they have elements that can be easily observed (e.g., church attendance as religious observance) and those that are not as readily observed (e.g., feeling closeness to God), and both represent primarily process-oriented phenomena, not fixed structural characteristics (e.g., religious denomination) (Dane, 2004).

Another concept that is important to clarify is spiritual pain (or suffering). Spiritual pain or suffering can be experienced by a person who is religious or nonreligious (who otherwise may have sense of transcendence) (Balduchi, 2010) and may manifest itself as symptoms in any area of a person's experience (e.g., physical, psychological, emotional, religious, or social) with characteristic descriptions and behaviors that help identify this form of suffering that threatens the core being of the person (Chochinov & Cann, 2005). Various dimensions of spiritual or existential suffering include loss of autonomy, control, and dignity, hopelessness, being a burden to others, and general despair (Chochinov & Cann, 2005).

Roles of Religion/Spirituality and Spiritual Care Interventions Near the End of Life

A person's religious faith and spirituality influence beliefs and efforts in finding meaning and purpose in the face of illness and death, decisions about health care, and experiences of distress and burden near the end of life (Phelps et al., 2009; Tarakeshwar et al., 2006). The one end-of-life topic on which several major religions have consensus, independent of denomination, is opposition to the euthanasia and assisted suicide. Most major religions, such as Buddhism, Christianity, Islam, and Judaism, prohibit these actions (Puchalski & O'Donnell, 2005). At the same time, most denominations or groups within these major religions take a more measured approach to the use of life-sustaining treatments and palliative care. For example, according to mainstream Christian beliefs, foregoing life-sustaining treatments is permissible when there is no reasonable hope of benefit or when treatment would impose excessive burden on the patient, family, or community. Similarly, Buddhist, Islamic, and Judaic teachings support withholding or withdrawing life-sustaining measures if the natural dying process is perceived to be prolonged without clear benefit or hope of recovery (Puchalski & O'Donnell, 2005).

However, some variability in preferences among people appears to exist across religions and within each religious group. For example, among Christians, fundamentalists are more likely to view faith as the most important source of coping and treatment during the end of life than those with less fundamental views (Vess, Arndt, Cox, Routledge, & Goldenberg, 2009). At the same time, Catholics are less likely than Protestants or other Christians to prefer life-sustaining treatment (Heeren, Menon, Raskin, & Ruskin, 2001); while, among followers of Judaism, more religiously observant practice is associated with a greater preference for the use of life-sustaining treatments such as feeding tubes (Sulmasy, 2006).

Spirituality and or religiosity also play an important role in maintaining the well-being of a person near the end of life (Steinhauser et al., 2000; Tarakeshwar et al., 2006). A systematic analysis of over 300 peer-reviewed journal articles on religion or spirituality and health found that spirituality is associated with better health, whereas religious distress can increase risk of death (Larson, Swyers, & McCullough, 1997). Another meta-analysis of terminally ill patients found that psycho-spiritual well-being was associated with increased coping with the symptoms of the illness, as well as an increased ability to find meaning from their experiences (Lin & Baur, 2003). Spiritual well-being also has been shown to improve quality of life and protect against depression, hopelessness, and desire for hastened death in patients with advanced cancer (Breitbart et al., 2000; McClain, Rosenfeld, & Breitbart, 2003). At the same time, spiritual distress has been shown to reduce quality of life near the end of life (Tarakeshwar et al., 2006).

There are interventions that aim to relieve spiritual or existential suffering by targeting various dimensions of spirituality such as meaning and purpose or hopelessness, burden to others, and suffering (Chochinov & Cann, 2005). Notable interventions that have shown promising results include Meaning-Centered Group Psychotherapy (Breitbart, 2002) and Dignity Therapy (Chochinov et al., 2005). A common feature of these interventions is that they may reduce existential or spiritual distress without having an explicit religious or faith-based focus (Chochinov & Cann, 2005).

Practice Recommendations

Practice recommendations for addressing spiritual distress by Rousseau (2000) suggest that counselors working with clients near the end of life need to attend to all four dimensions of care: physical, psychological, social and cultural, and spiritual and religious. Addressing physical symptoms is essential to providing spiritual care because uncontrolled, unnecessary physical pain and symptoms can greatly reduce quality of life and influence other dimensions of end-of-life experience including the spiritual (Rousseau, 2000). Counselors can help clients explore guilt, regret, forgiveness, and reconciliation, and encourage life review to evaluate and recognize purpose and meaning, facilitate religious expression, and encourage meditative practices promoting healing (e.g., finding solace, comfort, meaning, and purpose in the midst of suffering) rather than cure (Puchalski et al., 2009; Rousseau, 2000). An emphasis on hope also can be a powerful tool in the client's spiritual or religious system. By assessing the client's spiritual history, which provides a backdrop against which to understand the pressing spiritual questions that the dying client faces (Sulmasy, 2006), counselors can review the client's disclosures and investigate ways to realize their hopes, as well as be open-minded toward what the client is really trying to communicate. When counselors do not feel adequately trained and comfortable to address spiritual concerns of their clients, they can make referrals to professionals who have specialized training in spiritual care such as board-certified chaplains (Puchalski et al., 2009).

In order to connect with the client and listen to their most personal concerns, such as spiritual and existential suffering and fear, one of the most basic and yet essential practices for counselors is to explore their own assumptions, beliefs, and preparedness to work with clients around religious and spiritual issues. Five helpful questions offered by Merman (1992) include: whether life has meaning, what the patient's view of life after death is, what it means to "not be," what it means by "listening" to seriously ill and dying patients, and what it means to be honest with people who are dying. By exploring these questions, the counselor may become more aware of ambivalence, concerns, fear, and bias, and may learn to develop attitudes and skills to listen, respect, and mirror what his or her clients find important.

Another area of consideration pertains to the counselor's mental and or emotional state. In the therapeutic domain, there is a concept called "authentic presence" (Mahony, 1996). This is an attitude by which a person acknowledges, understands, and is confident in his or her actions to such an extent that she or he can naturally influence others to feel the same way. Similarly, practitioners who cultivate "present awareness," in which they practice being aware of what they are feeling and valuing in that moment, may allow them to gain a sense of what is important for the client at that present time (Craigie, 2010). In this way, practitioners may help clients feel calm in themselves as spiritual beings.

There are many variations of the perceived importance, and expression, of religious or spiritual identification. Hence, it is important for practitioners to be ready for different roles of religion and spirituality for individual clients and for unique individual expression and experience of spiritual, religious, and/or existential concerns and suffering among clients who are dying. For example, counselors need to recognize and respect diversity in the way different religious faith traditions express grief. Traditional Buddhist beliefs emphasize that it is most important to provide a quiet, meditative social environment for people who are dying, because of the belief that a dying person's last thoughts will influence how the individual will travel to the next life (Tsu, O'Conner, Bullwinkel, & Lee, 2009). In contrast, the religious expressions in some cultures in the African American community encourage the display of feelings because this shows love for the dying person (Cohen, McCannon, Edgman-Levitan, & Kormas, 2010). In sum, counselors need to look beyond religious cultural trappings and instead acknowledge, mirror, and validate the client and his or her family's sentiments.

CASE EXAMPLES

The following cases illustrate issues that affect communication, decision making, family support, grief, and religious and spiritual concerns of clients and families of different ethnic, cultural, religious, and spiritual backgrounds.

CASE 1: TAIFA AND ISAAC

Taifa was a 71-year-old African woman, who had emigrated from Nigeria to join her 48-year-old son and his family, and had been living in a Midwestern city for the past 20 years. Her English was limited, but she was able to make basic needs known. She has been recently diagnosed with advanced multiple sclerosis (MS). Taifa had been given a second social worker—the first was "fired" by Taifa's son, Isaac, for overlooking him and speaking directly to Taifa. Taifa, who identified as Muslim, was very deferent around Isaac, as was the custom of their household.

Despite the social worker's attempts, Taifa agreed with her son and refused to fill out the paperwork for a power of attorney or living will, stating that where they came from in Africa, they did not fill out paperwork that prepared one for death. In turn, Taifa attempted to defer to the physicians for medical decision making, saying she trusted the "healers" in making the right choice for her. Despite the fact that there was no official power of attorney form, her medical team became accustomed to allowing Isaac to direct care decisions on behalf of Taifa.

As Taifa's condition worsened and placement in a nursing home was considered, the social worker tried to gain trust by holding conversations with Isaac and Taifa to explore what was needed to make her and her family feel at peace in this situation. In her final weeks, Taifa received comfort measures in her home, and only shortly before death was she placed in a hospital hospice wing to treat her complicated medical needs. Not long after the time of death, at the behest of family, the social worker asked the hospital for permission for the body to remain in the hospital room while her family and hospital staff participated in an after-death ritual of washing the body. The social worker followed up with bereavement counseling for Isaac, and was informed that Taifa's cremated remains were shipped to their home in Africa. Isaac commented that having her remains buried at their ancestral home helped him feel closure to his mother's end-of-life story.

Implications of this story include the importance of flexibility in considering a patient and her or his family's culture in problem solving. In this case, Taifa valued family harmony was more important than individual autonomy, and the social worker acknowledged Taifa's values by respecting her son as the head of household and main caregiver. The social worker's conduct of relating to the son as the decision maker in turn allowed him to "soften," and thus trust in their relationship. Further, the social worker also acknowledged culture by asking the hospital to allow for the family's need to conduct an after-death ritual.

CASE 2: WYATT

Wyatt is a 43-year-old Mexican American man who lived on the West coast. After years of struggling with kidney disease, he was diagnosed with a progressive form of renal failure. He had a long-time social worker through Medicaid. He often commented about how "God's got my back," and "God will heal me." At that time, Wyatt was still very mobile and active, and though he knew what his diagnosis could lead to, he did not let go of his belief that he would be able to heal from his present condition.

A month later, Wyatt's medical condition had advanced considerably. He was no longer as physically mobile, expressed feeling hopeless, and was exhausted by the continuous rounds of dialysis and medications that were used to moderate his symptoms. Wyatt's dialysis team contacted the social worker about Wyatt's depressive behaviors. Wyatt confided to his social worker that the biggest problem in his life was his growing doubt about his faith in God. He admitted he felt very discouraged that in spite of all the prayers from his family, his condition is not improving; in fact it was getting worse.

In successive visits, the social worker carefully shifted the discussion from God to his feelings about the loss brought on by his illness. When prompted about his needs, Wyatt said his main need was for a reprieve from his physical symptoms. Because that was not always under his control, the social worker encouraged Wyatt to explore ways in which he could seek absolution in areas of his life over which he did have more control. After that discussion, Wyatt decided to try to address the troubled relationships in his life.

The last time the social worker visited with Wyatt, he was bed-bound and appeared very frail. Wyatt also commented that he continued to doubt his religion. His tenor was different from what the social worker had heard before. He said he no longer dwelled on his faith the way he used to, because he had only so much energy, which he chose to spend on those he cared about most.

This case study illustrates the importance of deep listening. The social worker helped the client shift his perspective toward the here and now, which can become more relevant during the loss of meaning sometimes experienced in the dying process.

CONCLUSION

In an increasingly multiracial, multiethnic, and multicultural society, where most deaths occur later in life, it is important for counselors to have a comprehensive, holistic approach to understanding and working effectively with each client and family system within their own unique physical, psychological, social, cultural, and religious/spiritual contexts. Keeping in mind the crucial fact that no one experiences dying and death in the same way, counselors can work to broaden their understanding and develop respect and appreciation for the complex interplay of various factors that influence the end-of-life experiences of clients and their families.

CLINICAL PEARL

Major Areas of Assessment When Counseling Clients and Their Families and Support Systems Near the End of Life

Most practice guidelines for palliative care and theoretical frameworks on end-of-life care identify at least four major dimensions of end-of-life experiences: physical, psychological, social and cultural, and spiritual/religious dimensions. Below is a list of potential essential areas of assessment and intervention for diverse clients and their families near the end of life.

- *Physical Dimension*
  - Functional trajectories, associated care demands, and transitions in care settings (e.g., home, nursing homes, hospitals, in-patient hospice facilities)
  - Physical distress: physical pain and nonpain symptoms (e.g., nausea, fatigue, weakness)
- *Psychological Dimension*
  - Fear of dying, sadness, grief, and dignity and psychiatric illnesses (e.g., anxiety, depression, hopelessness, suicide ideation)
- *Social and Cultural Dimension*
  - Key demographic characteristics (e.g., age, race/ethnicity)
  - Socioeconomic resources (e.g., education, health literacy, economic resources, social resources such as family caregivers, friends, and neighbors, English proficiency)
  - Cultural identity (e.g., acculturation level)
  - Cultural beliefs regarding communication and decision making about illness and treatments (e.g., illness explanation, attitudes toward talking about death and dying, help-seeking behavior, role of traditional healing methods, how and who makes the final decision)
  - Personal experience with illness, access to health care, discrimination, relationship with health care providers
  - Family well-being (e.g., grief, sadness, depression, spiritual, and religious concerns) and caregiving capacities and concerns (e.g.,

(continued)

CLINICAL PEARL (*continued*)

caregiving burden and stress, physical health, concerns about communication and decision making, education, training, and counseling support needs)
- *Spiritual/Religious Dimension*
  ○ Religious beliefs about end-of-life issues (e.g., life-sustaining treatments), religious coping (e.g., prayer) and support (e.g., church), spiritual well-being and concerns (e.g., meaning, purpose, hope, concerns about loss of autonomy, control, and dignity, being a burden on others, despair)

REFERENCES

Allen, J. Y., Hilgeman, M. M., & Allen, R. S. (2010). Prospective end-of-life treatment decisions and perceived vulnerability: Future time left to live and memory self-efficacy. *Aging and Mental Health, 15,* 122–131.

Azoulay, E., Chevret, S., Leleu, G., Pochard, F., Barboteu, M., Adrie, C., ... Schlemmer, B. (2000). Half the families of intensive care unit patients experience inadequate communication with physicians. *Critical Care Medicine, 28,* 3044–3049.

Balduchi, L. (2010). Beyond quality of life: The meaning of death and suffering in palliative care. *Asian Pacific Journal of Cancer Prevention, 11,* 41–44.

Bito, S., Matsumura, S., Singer, M. K., Meredith, L. S., Fukuhara, S., & Wenger, N. S. (2007). Acculturation and end-of-life decision making: Comparison of Japanese and Japanese American focus groups. *Bioethics, 21,* 251–262.

Blackhall, L. J., Frank, G., Murphy, S. T., Michel, V., Palmer, J. M., & Azen, S. P. (1999). Ethnicity and attitudes towards life sustaining technology. *Social Science & Medicine, 48*(12), 1779–1789.

Blackhall, L. J., Murphy, S. T., Frank, G., Michel, V., Palmer, J. M., & Azen, S. (1995). Ethnicity and attitudes toward patient autonomy. *Journal of the American Medical Association, 274,* 820–825.

Block, S. D. (2001). Psychological considerations, growth, and transcendence at the end of life: The art of the possible. *Journal of the American Medical Association, 285,* 2898–2905.

Boelen, P. A., & Prigerson, H. G. (2007). The influence of symptoms of prolonged grief disorder, depression, and anxiety on quality of life bereaved adults: A prospective study. *European Archives of Psychiatry and Clinical Neuroscience, 257,* 444–452.

Bonanno, G. A., & Kaltman, S. (2001). The varieties of grief experience. *Clinical Psychology Review, 21,* 705–734.

Borum, M. L., Lynn, J., & Zhong, Z. (2000). The effects of patient race on outcomes in seriously ill patients in SUPPORT: An overview of economic impact, medical intervention, and end-of-life decisions. *Journal of the American Geriatrcis Society, 48,* S194–S198.

Bowman, K. (2004). What are the limits of bioethics in a culturally pluralistic societ? *Journal of Law and Medical Ethics, 32,* 664–669.

Breen, C. M., Abernethy, A. P., Abbott, K. H., & Tulsky, J. A. (2001). Conflict associated with decisions to limit life-sustaining treatment in intensive care units *Journal of General Internal Medicine, 16,* 283–289.

Breitbart, W. (2002). Spirituality and meaning in supportive care: Spirituality- and meaning-centered group psychotherapy interventions in advanced cancer. *Cancer, 10,* 272–280.

Breitbart, W., Rosenfeld, B., Gibson, C., Kramer, M., Li, Y., Tomarken, A., ... Schuster, M. (2010). Impact of treatment for depression on desire for hastened death in patients with advanced AIDS. *Psychosomatics, 51,* 98–105.

Breitbart, W., Rosenfeld, B., Pessin, H., Kaim, M., Funesti-Esch, J., Galietta, M., ... Brescia, R. (2000). Depression, hopelessness, and desire for death in terminally ill patients with cancer. *Journal of the American Medical Association, 284,* 2907–2911.

Burrs, F. A. (1995). The African American experience: Breaking the barriers to Hospices. *Hospice Journal, 10,* 15–18.

Carrese, J. A., & Rhodes, L. A. (1995). Western bioethics on the Navajo Reservation: Benefit or harm? *Journal of the American Medical Association, 274,* 826–829.

Centers for Disease Control and Prevention. (1993). Use of race and ethnicity in public health surveillance: Summary of the CDC/ATSDR Workshop. *Morbidity and Mortality Weekly Report (Vol. No. RR-10).* Atlanta: Author.

Chochinov, H. M., & Cann, B. J. (2005). Interventions to enhance the spiritual aspects of dying. *Journal of Palliative Medicine, 8,* s-103–s-115.

Chochinov, H. M., Hack, T., Hassard, T., Kristjanson, L., McClement, S., & Harlos, M. (2005). Dignity therapy: A novel psychotherapeutic intervention for patients nearing death. *Journal of Clinical Oncology, 23,* 5520–5525.

Christakis, N. A., & Lamont, E. B. (2000). Extent and determinants of error in doctors' prognoses in terminally ill patients: Prospective cohort study. *British Medical Journal, 320,* 469–472.

Cohen, H., Thomas, C., & Williamson, C. (2008). Religion and spirituality as defined by older adults. *Journal of Gerontological Social Work, 51,* 284–297.

Cohen, M. J., McCannon, J. B., Edgman-Levitan, S., & Kormos, W. A. (2010). Exploring attitudes toward advance care directives in two diverse settings. *Journal of Palliative Medicine, 13,* 1427–1432.

Craigie, F. C. (2010). *Positive spirituality in health care.* Minneapolis, MN: Mill City Press.

Dane, B. (2004). Integrating spirituality and religion. In J. Berzoff, & P. R. Silverman (Eds.), *Living with dying: A handbook for end-of-life health care practitioners* (pp. 424–438). New York: Columbia University Press.

Ditto, P. H., Hawkins, N. A., & Pizarro, D. A. (2005). Imagining the end of life: On the psychology of advance medical decision making. *Motivation and Emotion, 29,* 481–503.

Dumont, S., Turgeon, J., Allard, P., Gagnon, P., Charbonneau, C., & Vezina, L. (2006). Caring for a loved one with advanced cancer: Determinants of psychological distress in family caregivers. *Journal of Palliative Medicine, 9,* 912–921.

Ebell, M. H., Doukas, D. J., & Simth, M. A. (1991). The do-not-resuscitate order: A comparison of physician and patient preferences and decision-making. *The American Journal of Medicine, 91*, 255–260.

Egede, L. E. (2006). Race, ethnicity, and disparities in health care. *Journal of General Internal Medicine, 21*, 667–669.

Engel, S. E., Kiely, D. K., & Mitchell, S. L. (2006). Satisfaction with end-of-life care for nursing home residents with advanced dementia. *Journal of the American Geriatrics Society, 54*, 1567–1572.

Ersek, M., Kawaga-Singer, M., Barnes, D., Blackhall, L. J., & Koenig, B. A. (1998). Multicultural considerations in the use of advance directives. *Oncology Nursing Forum, 25*, 1683–1690.

Gallup. (2008). *Americans believe religion is losing clout*. Retrieved March 7, 2012, from http://www.gallup.com/poll/113533/Americans-Believe-Religion-Losing-Clout.aspx

Gallup. (2011). *Religion in the United States*. Retrieved March 2, 2012, from http://www.gallup.com/poll/151760/Christianity-Remains-Dominant-Religion-United-states.aspx

Gebara, J., & Tashjian, H. (2006). End-of-life practices at a Lebanese hospital: Courage or knowledge? *Journal of Transcultural Nursing, 17*, 381–388.

Gessert, C. E., Forbes, S., & Bern-Klug, M. (2000). Planning end-of-life care for patients with dementia: Roles of families and health professionals. *Omega, 42*, 273–291.

Glaser, B. G., & Strauss, A. L. (1968). *Time for dying*. Chicago: Aldine Publishing.

Gott, M., Barnes, S., Parker, C., Payne, S., Seamark, D., Gariballa, S., & Small, N. (2007). Dying trajectories in heart failure. *Palliative Medicine, 21*, 95–99.

Hanson, L. C., Danis, M., & Garrett, J. (1997). What is wrong with end-of-life care? Opinions of bereaved family members. *Journal of the American Geriatrics Society, 45*, 1339–1344.

Heeren, O., Menon, A. S., Raskin, A., & Ruskin, P. (2001). Religion and end of life treatment preferences among geriatric patients. *International Journal of Geriatric Psychiatry, 16*, 203–208.

Imperato, P. J., Nenner, R. P., & Will, T. O. (1996). Radical prostatectomy: Lower rates among African-American men. *Journal of the National Medical Association, 88*, 589–594.

Intrator, O., Zinn, J., & Mor, V. (2004). Nursing home characteristics and potentially preventable hospitalizations of long-stay residents. *Journal of the American Geriatrcis Society, 52*, 1730–1736.

Johnstone, M.-J., & Kanitsaki, O. (2009). Ethics and advance care planning in a culturally diverse society. *Journal of Transcultural Nursing, 20*, 405–416.

Kaut, K. (2006). End of life assessment within a holistic bio-psycho-social-spiritual framework. In J. L. Werth, Jr., & D. Blevins (Eds.), *Psychosocial issues near the end of life: A resource for professional care providers* (pp. 111–136). Washington, DC: American Psychological Association.

Keovilay, L., Rasbreidge, L., & Kemp, C. (2000). Cambodian and Laotian health beliefs and practices related to the end of life. *Journal of Hospice and Palliative Care Nursing, 2*, 143–151.

Kochanek, K. D., Xu, J. Q., Murphy, S. L., Miniño, A. M., & Kung, H. (2011). Deaths: Preliminary data for 2009. *National vital statistics reports (Vol. 59)*. Hyattsville, MD: National Center for Health Statistics.

Krakauer, E. L., Crenner, C., & Fox, K. (2002). Barriers to optimum end-of-life care for minority patients. *Journal of the American Geriatrics Society, 50,* 182–190.

Kramer, B. J., Boelk, A. Z., & Auer, C. (2006). Family conflict at the end of life: Lessons learned in a model program for vulnerable older adults. *Journal of Palliative Medicine, 9,* 791–801.

Kwak, J., Allen, J. Y., & Haley, W. E. (2011). Advance care planning and end-of-life decision making. In P. Dilworth-Anderson, & M. H. Palmer (Eds.), *Annual review of gerontology and geriatrics: Pathways through the transitions of care for older adults* (Vol. 31, pp. 143–165). New York: Springer Publishing.

Kwak, J., & Haley, W. E. (2005). Current research findings on end-of-life decision making among racially or ethnically diverse groups. *The Gerontologist, 45*(5), 634–641.

Kwak, J., Haley, W. E., & Chiriboga, D. A. (2008). Racial differences in hospice use and in-hospital death among Medicare and Medicaid dual-eligible nursing home residents. *The Gerontologist, 48,* 32–41.

Kwak, J., Salmon, J. R., Acquaviva, K., Brandt, K., & Egan, K. (2007). Benefits of training family caregivers on experiences of closure during end-of-life care. *Journal of Pain and Symptom Management, 33,* 434–445.

Larson, D. B., Swyers, J. P., & McCullough, M. E. (1997). *Scientific research on spirituality and health: A consensus report.* Rockville, MD: National Institute for Healthcare Research.

Levine, C., Halper, D., Peist, A., & Gould, D. A. (2010). Bridging troubled waters: Family caregivers, transitions, and long-term care. *Health Affairs, 29,* 116–124.

Lin, H., & Baur, S. (2003). Psycho-spiritual well-being in patients with advanced cancer: An integrative review of the literature. *Journal of Advanced Nursing, 44,* 69–80.

Lunney, J. R., Lynn, J., Foley, D. J., Lipson, S., & Guralnik, J. M. (2003). Patterns of functional decline at the end of life. *Journal of the American Medical Association, 289,* 2387–2392.

Lunney, J. R., Lynn, J., & Hogan, C. (2002). Profiles of older medicare decedents. *Journal of the American Geriatrics Society, 50*(6), 1108–1112.

Mahony, M. (1996). Authentic presence and compassionate wisdom: The art of Jim Bugental. *Journal of Humanistic Psychology, 36,* 58–66.

McClain, C. S., Rosenfeld, B., & Breitbart, W. (2003). Effect of spiritual well-being on end-of-life despair in terminally ill patients. *Lancet, 361,* 1603–1607.

McGrath, P. (2003). Religiosity and the challenge of terminal illness. *Death Studies, 27,* 881–899.

Merman, A. (1992). Spiritual aspects of death and dying. *Yale Journal of Biology and Medicine, 65,* 137–142.

Mezey, M., Dubler, N., Mitty, E., & Brody, A. A. (2002). What impact do setting and transitions have on the quality of life at the end of life and the quality of the dying process? *The Gerontologist, 42,* 54–67.

Murphy, S. T., Palmer, J. M., Azen, S., Frank, G., Michel, V., & Blackhall, L. J. (1996). Ethnicity and advance directives. *Journal of Law and Medical Ethics, 24,* 108–117.

National Consensus Project for Quality Palliative Care. (2009). *Clinical practice guidelines for quality palliative care.* Pittsburgh: Author.

Payne, R. (2001). Palliative care for African-Americans and other vulnerable populations: Access and equality issues. In K. M. Foley, & H. Gleband (Eds.), *Improving palliative care for cancer* (pp. 153–160). Washington, DC: National Academies Press.

Phelps, A. C., Maciejewski, P., Nilsson, M., Balboni, T., Wright, A., Paulk, M., ... Prigerson, H. G. (2009) Religious coping and use of intensive lifeprolonging care near death in patients with advanced cancer. *Journal of the American Medical Association, 301*, 1140–1147.

Phillips, R. S., Hamel, M. B., Teno, J. M., Bellamy, P., Broste, S. K., Califf, R. M., ... Connors, A. F. (1996). Race, resource use, and survival in seriously ill hospitalized adults. *Journal of General Internal Medicine, 11*, 387–396.

Pickens, N. D., O'Reilly, K. R., & Sharp, K. C. (2010). Holding on to normalcy and overshadowed needs: Family caregiving at end of life. *Canadian Journal of Occupational Therapy—Revue Canadienne d Ergotherapie, 77*, 234–240.

Puchalski, C., Ferrell, B., Virani, R., Otis-Green, S., Baird, P., Bull, J., ... Sulmasy, D. (2009). Improving the quality of spiritual care as a dimension of palliative care: The Report of the Consensus Conference. *Journal of Palliative Medicine, 12*, 885–904.

Puchalski, C. M., & O'Donnell, E. (2005). Religious and spiritual beliefs in end of life care: How major religions view death and dying. *Techniques in Regional Anesthesia and Pain Management, 9*, 114–121.

Reese, D. J., Ahern, R. E., Nair, S., Schorock, J. D. O., & Warren-Weath, C. (1999). Hospice access and use by African Americans: Addressing cultural and institutional barriers through participatory action research. *Social Work, 44*, 549–559.

Rio, N. D. (2004). Framework for multicultural end-of-life care: Enhancing social work practice. In J. Berzoff, & P. R. Silverman (Eds.), *Living with dying: A handbook for end-of-life health care practitioners* (pp. 439–461). New York: Columbia University Press.

Rousseau, P. (2000). Spirituality and the dying patient. *Journal of Clinical Oncology, 18*, 2000–2002.

Salmon, J. R., Kwak, J., Acquaviva, K., Brandt, K., & Egan, K. (2005). Transformative aspects of caregiving at life's end. *Journal of Pain and Symptom Management, 22*, 188–194.

Searight, H. R., & Gafford, J. (2005). It's like playing with your destiny: Bosnian immigrants' views of advance directives and end of life decision making. *Journal of Immigrant Health, 7*, 195–203.

Sharma, G., Freeman, J., Zhang, D., & Goodwin, J. S. (2009). Continuity of care and intensive care unit use at the end of life. *Archives of Internal Medicine, 169*, 81–86.

Shear, M. K., Simon, N., Wall, M., Zisook, S., Neimeyer, R., Duan, N., ... Keshaviah, A. (2011). Complicated grief and related bereavement issues for DSM-5. *Depression and Anxiety, 28*, 103–117.

Smedly, B. D., Stith, A. Y., & Nelson, A. R. (2003). *Unequal treatment: Confronting racial and ethnic disparities in health care*. Washington, DC: National Academies Press.

Steinhauser, K. E., Christakis, N. A., Clipp, E. C., McNeilly, M., McIntyre, L., & Tulsky, J. A. (2000). Factors considered important at the end of life by patients, family, physicians, and other care providers. *Journal of the American Medical Association, 284*, 2476–2482.

Sulmasy, D. (2006). Spiritual issues in the care of dying patients: " ... It's okay between me and God". *Journal of the American Medical Association, 296,* 1385–1392.

SUPPORT Principal Investigators. (1995). A controlled trial to improve care for seriously ill hospitalized patients. The study to understand prognoses and preferences for outcomes and risks of treatments (SUPPORT). *Journal of the American Medical Association, 274,* 1591–1598.

Tarakeshwar, N., Vanderwerker, L. C., Paulk, E., Pearce, M. J., Kasl, S. V., & Prigerson, H. G. (2006). Religious coping is associated with the quality of life of patients with advanced cancer. *Journal of Palliative Medicine, 9,* 646–657.

Teno, J. M., Clarridge, B. R., Casey, V., Welch, L. C., Wetle, T., Shield, R., & Mor, V. (2004). Family perspectives on end-of-life care at the last place of care. *Journal of the American Medical Association, 291,* 88–93.

Tilden, V. P., Tolle, S., Drach, L., & Hickman, S. (2002). Measurement of quality of care and quality of life at the end of life. *The Gerontologist, 42*(Special Issue III), 71–80.

Tsu, C., O'Conner, M., Bullwinkel, V., & Lee, S. (2009). Understandings of death and dying for people of Chinese origin. *Death Studies, 33,* 153–174.

Unruh, A. M., Versnel, J., & Kerr, N. (2002). Spirituality unplugged: A review of commonalities and contentions, and a resolution. *Canadian Journal of Occupational Therapy, 69,* 5–19.

U.S. Administration on Aging. (2010). *Projected future growth of the older population: By race and Hispanic origin: 2000–2050.* Retrieved March 2, 2012, from http://www.aoa.gov/AoARoot/Aging_Statistics/future_growth/future_growth.aspx#hispanic

U.S. Census Bureau. (2004). *U.S. interim projections by age, sex, race, and Hispanic origin.* Retrieved March 2, 2012, 2012, from http://www.census.gov/ipc/www/usinterimproj/

U.S. Department of Health and Human Services Office of Minority Health. (1999). *Assuring cultural competence in health care: Recommendations for national standards and outcomes-focused research agenda.* Washington, DC: U.S. Government Printing Office.

Vess, M., Arndt, J., Cox, C. R., Routledge, C., & Goldenberg, J. L. (2009). Exploring the existential function of religion: The effect of religious fundamentalism and mortality salience on faith-based medical refusals. *Journal of Personality and Social Psychology, 97,* 334–350.

Waters, C. M. (2001). Understanding and supporting African Americans' perspectives of end-of-life planning and decision making. *Qualitative Health Research, 11,* 385–398.

Weitzen, S., Teno, J. M., Fennell, M., & Mor, V. (2003). Factors associated with site of death: A national study of where people die. *Medical Care, 4,* 323–335.

World Health Orgnization. (2004). *Better palliative care for older people.* Retrieved October 10, 2004, from http://www.euro.who.int/document/E82933.pdf

3

Advance Directives: Planning for the End of Life

REBECCA S. ALLEN, MORGAN K. EICHORST, AND JOANN OLIVER

Advance care planning is a general term encompassing processes by which an individual communicates his or her preferences for future end-of-life care in an informal (e.g., discussions) or formal (e.g., advance directives such as living wills or health care power of attorney, do-not-resuscitate orders, do-not-hospitalize orders) manner to others such as health care providers (HCPs), family members (e.g., relatives by blood or marriage and fictive kin), and members of social support systems (e.g., clergy, friends). Since the Patient Self Determination Act (PSDA) (Omnibus Budget Reconciliation Act of 1990) became effective on December 1, 1991, health care institutions such as hospitals, home health care agencies, nursing homes, and hospices that receive federal funds such as Medicare have been required to "educate" potential patients about their rights to make decisions about their own health care. The specific requirements of the PSDA are that individuals: (1) have the right to facilitate their own health care decisions; (2) have the right to accept or refuse medical treatments; and (3) have the right to execute an advance directive. The PSDA also requires that institutions inquire whether the individual has an advance directive and make note of the existence of such a document in their medical records, as well as educate staff and affiliates about an individual's rights to engage in advance care planning and to execute advance directives.

The completion of advance directives and engagement in advance care planning prior to a health crisis has been advocated, but reimbursement for physicians or other HCPs to counsel patients about their rights was omitted from the 2010 Affordable Care Act, Medicare wellness visits, and new CMS practice guidelines because of public concern regarding "death panels" (Tinetti, 2012). Individuals and their family members or HCPs tend to delay consideration of preferences for end-of-life medical treatments (Allen, Haley, Roff, Schmid, & Bergman, 2006; Bailey et al., 2012). Moreover, medical providers are not accurate with prognostication, sometimes misestimating an individual's time left to live by a factor of up to 5 (Chow et al., 2011; Christakis & Lamont, 2000; Stiel et al., 2009). Discussions regarding the potential of death tend to occur very late in the disease process, if such discussions occur at all (Bailey et al., 2012; Guo et al., 2010; SUPPORT Principal Investigators, 1995; Tschann, Kaufman, & Micco, 2003). Clearly, a role for clinicians across disciplines exists in facilitating the effective and therapeutic discussion of advance care plans and the potential completion of advance directives. Clinicians such as social workers, nurses, psychologists, and behaviorists can assist individuals with advanced, chronic illness, their HCPs, and family members in the consideration of physical, mental, and spiritual quality of life issues that may clarify goals of care and treatment preferences near the end of life.

This chapter focuses on individual characteristics associated with advance directive completion, shared decision making, racial/ethnic differences and disparities, environmental context of decisions (e.g., community, long-term, acute, and critical care), and interventions to improve the ongoing process of advance care planning and the completion of advance directives. Two case studies are provided for consideration. The chapter ends with implications for practice and potential avenues for future research.

CHARACTERISTICS PREDICTING COMPLETION OF ADVANCE DIRECTIVES

Factors that influence completion of advance directives include age, individual attitudes, cultural beliefs, and trust in HCPs, and health status, including receipt of care in differing types of health care settings (Jones, Moss, & Harris-Kojetin, 2011; Phipps et al., 2003; Rosnick & Reynolds, 2003). Jones and colleagues (2011) reported data from the 2004 National Nursing Home Survey and the 2007 National Home and Hospice Care Survey, showing that living wills and do-not-resuscitate (DNR) orders were the most common types of advance directives. A living will is a legal document created based on state law that makes an individual's wishes regarding life-sustaining or life-prolonging medical care known in advance of medical crisis. Moreover, prevalence rates of advance directives were higher among individuals receiving any type of long-term care (e.g., home health care, skilled nursing home care, hospice care) in comparison with the overall U.S. adult population (Jones et al., 2011).

In response to media attention regarding health care reform, Silveira, Kim, and Langa (2010) examined proxy-reported data of community-dwelling individuals ($N = 3,746$) who had died across 6 years in the Health and Retirement Study (2000–2006). The proxies were interviewed within 2 years of the participants' deaths and were asked whether the participant had completed a living will or durable power of attorney for health care, maintained decision-making capacity, and experienced medical issues that required decision making at the end of life. Proxies reported that 42.5% of prior Health and Retirement Study participants experienced medical situations that required decision making and that 70.3% of these individuals lacked decision-making capacity at the required time. Nearly 68% of individuals who lacked decisional capacity possessed advance directives. Regarding the match between care preferences and receipt of care, 83.2% of individuals who requested limited care and 97.1% of those who requested comfort care received care consistent with their preferences. Among the 10 individuals who requested all care possible, only five received it (Silveira et al., 2010).

Downar and colleagues (2011) conducted a qualitative analysis of semi-structured interviews and achieved conceptual saturation with 44 patients who had clearly requested a specific type of end-of-life care (i.e., DNR or full code) after discussions with their medical team. Using a grounded theory approach, they found that patients in the DNR group were much older, had similar comorbidities, were more familiar with the subject of resuscitation discussions, and reported a more positive experience with such discussions than did full code patients. Although not directly stated by these authors, the individuals who requested DNR may also have been more educated about the benefits and risks of resuscitation, or had greater health literacy. Most full code patients reported they would not want an extended period on life support and would not want life support under conditions of poor quality of life. Full code and DNR patients understood resuscitation differently, with DNR patients describing resuscitation in graphic terms of suffering and DNR as natural. Full code patients' descriptions were more general and focused on resuscitation as a means of restoring life.

Regarding characteristics of individuals with a DNR order, Brink, Smith, and Kitson (2008) examined the medical records of 470 home health care clients in Canada. They found that a preference to die at home, close proximity to death, daily incontinence, sleep problems, and an individual's acceptance of the nearness of death were associated with having a DNR order. Chang and colleagues (2010) conducted a prospective correlational study in Taiwan of critically ill patients ($N = 202$) with and without DNR orders in ICUs to compare the kinds of end-of-life treatments received. Similar to data reported in U.S. intensive care units (ICUs), they found that nearly 66% of patients had a DNR order. In the last 48 hours of life, patients with a DNR order were significantly less likely to receive life-supporting therapies. Predictors of having a DNR order included older age, being unmarried, the presence of an adult child as a surrogate decision maker, a perceived inability to survive discharge from an ICU, and longer length of stay in the ICU.

In summary, individuals who possess advance directives tend to perceive a sense of personal vulnerability (i.e., older age, poor health status, acceptance of the nearness of death) and have a preference for independent and autonomous decision making. Given these characteristics, clinicians across disciplines can identify individual clients that may be open to discussions about advance directives. Understanding the characteristics of typical individuals with advance directives can also assist the clinician in creating therapeutic interventions for others who do not fit this pattern. Potential interventions for vulnerable populations will be discussed in a later section of this chapter.

Personal Perceptions of Vulnerability

Individuals with advanced, chronic illness and in receipt of long-term care in the community or residential care settings may experience a sense of vulnerability that encourages advance care planning discussions and completion of advance directives. Among a community-dwelling sample consisting of approximately equal numbers of older Caucasian and African American adults, Allen, Hilgeman, and Allen (2011) found that individuals with more expansive perceptions of time left to live and those with better perceived memory (lower perceived memory change and higher perceived memory capacity) reported a greater desire for life-sustaining medical treatments when presented with hypothetical illness scenarios. In other words, older individuals who perceived less time to live and memory problems were more likely to forego future life-sustaining treatments. Another study found that even among adults aged 64 to 65, hospitalization within the last year was associated with an increased likelihood of having engaged in various types of advance care planning (Carr & Khodyakov, 2007). The results of these studies emphasize the variability in individual's self-evaluations and how these self-evaluations might influence the advance care planning process. Clinicians should be aware of these differences and seek to understand the individual client in an effort to present advance care planning options in a culturally appropriate and efficacious way. Although little is known about racial/ethnic or cultural variation in individual perceptions of vulnerability, much is known about racial/ethnic variation in advance care planning and completion of advance directives.

Racial/Ethnic Differences and Disparities

End-of-life planning involves important decisions, and racial and ethnic cultural differences play a role in how and when treatment decisions are made. Ethnic minorities compose about a third of the United States population

(United States Census Bureau, 2001). Culture is defined as similarities in values, beliefs, and behaviors that a group of people have in common that is transmitted across generations. According to the literature, there have been significant differences in advance care planning identified by race and ethnicity (Crawley et al., 2000; Hopp & Duffy, 2000; Krakauer, Crenner, & Fox, 2002; Kwak & Haley, 2005). Based upon these differences, assistance with and approaches to end-of-life care or planning may vary considerably. For example, African American and Hispanic patients are less likely to have an advance care plan or know about advance directives (Kwak & Haley, 2005; Perkins, Geppert, Gonzales, Cortez, & Hazuda, 2002; Smith et al., 2008).

Racial and ethnic minorities are less likely to use hospice care, but more likely to receive hospital-based and life-sustaining medical interventions such as resuscitation and cardiac conversion (i.e., a medical procedure in which an abnormally fast heart rate or cardiac arrhythmia is converted into normal rhythm), mechanical ventilation, and artificial nutrition in comparison to Caucasians (Crawley et al., 2000; Hanchate, Kronman, Young-Xu, Ash, & Emanuel, 2009). Smith and colleagues (2008) reported that Black and Hispanic patients were less likely to consider themselves terminally ill and were more likely to want aggressive treatment. These findings were consistent with a previous study that included 50 African American and 27 Caucasian patients where more than 50% of the African American patients wanted life-sustaining treatment in a case example involving chronic conditions and "brain death," compared to only 11% of the Caucasians preferring these measures (Bayer, Mallinger, Krishnan, & Shields, 2006).

African Americans' history of health care discrimination and unequal care may play a vital role in their reluctance to formally address end-of-life care, such as low use of hospice care (Crawley et al., 2000). For example, African Americans are less likely to accept DNR orders and are more likely to change from DNR to more aggressive levels of care (Searight & Gafford, 2005). Aggressive medical care that is provided to a person who is dying is defined as care and treatment that provides a means of prolonging life (Searight & Gafford, 2005). A possible explanation for this pattern of results can be found in studies demonstrating that minorities may perceive palliative care and DNR orders as less than optimal care (e.g., Cardenas-Turanzas, Gaeta, Ashoori, Price, & Nates, 2011).

Although some studies report that African Americans prefer more aggressive care at the end of life than Caucasians, race may not be the only factor of influence. Health literacy or the need for enhanced information or patient education regarding the risks and benefits of end-of-life medical treatments may be important issues for clinicians to consider (Allen, Allen, Hilgeman, & DeCoster, 2008; O'Connor et al., 2007; Volandes et al., 2008). For example, Volandes and colleagues (2008) reported that the differences exhibited by African Americans and Caucasians in treatment preferences were nonexistent once the experimenters controlled for varying levels of health literacy, suggesting that more complex variables could account for the differences. Furthermore, there were no differences whatsoever in treatment preferences for either racial group and for the varying levels of health literacy once participants were shown a 2-minute video (vs. a verbal description) about advanced dementia (Volandes et al., 2008). Using a different decision aid and different illness scenarios, Allen and colleagues (2008) found that provision of enhanced information regarding hypothetical end-of-life medical treatments reduced decisional conflict among both African American and Caucasian older adults; however, differing patterns of treatment preference were still found. Hence, clinicians may be able to assist HCPs in choosing decision aids that provide needed information to patients regarding specific treatment options in a universally accessible and culturally competent way. Knowledge and awareness of racial and ethnic differences are imperative. Individuals with advanced, chronic illness and their families are vulnerable and will require culturally appropriate and sensitive care. Clinicians must be keenly aware and engage in culturally appropriate levels of disclosure in efforts to address issues involving advance directives and end-of-life care with their clients and colleagues in order to facilitate the most effective and shared decision making. Decision making may be an autonomous process or one that is shared with HCPs or with family members; this is the topic of the next section.

SHARED DECISION MAKING

Individuals vary in their desire for the involvement of family in the advance care planning and decision-making process, but even if they prefer the involvement of family, a familial proxy holds no legal status under current laws of informed consent unless the individual in question has been determined to be incompetent (Allen & Shuster, 2002). The purpose of advance care planning, however, is to document the treatment preferences of healthy and competent individuals well in advance of medical crisis. Data from the Wisconsin Longitudinal Study (Moorman, 2011) indicated that over three-quarters of relatively healthy Caucasian Midwesterners who were high school graduates reported that they would prefer to make decisions independently, and that they would choose to have their wishes followed strictly. Notably, this population may be more empowered with higher health literacy and more desire for independence than an older minority population, who might prefer a shared decision-making model.

Although advance care planning and the completion of advance directives can be considered a patient-centered preventive health behavior, the U.S. Preventive Services Task Force (USPSTF; www.ahrq.gov/clinic/uspstfix.htm), created in 1984, has been relatively silent on the topic. Recent public outcry in reaction to the "death panel" discussion has created a policy movement away from advance care planning (Tinetti, 2012). The USPSTF is an independent group of national experts in prevention and evidence-based medicine that works to improve the health of all Americans by making evidence-based recommendations about clinical preventive services such as screenings, counseling services, or preventive medications. The USPSTF, rather than stating recommendations regarding advance care planning, has instead focused on the detection of dementia in primary care settings and noted the potential benefits of early detection of dementia in promoting advance care planning and completion of advance directives. Identification of individuals at risk for loss of capacity may help HCPs engage individuals and families in advance care planning and the completion of advance directives (Boustani, Peterson, Hanson, Harris, & Lohr, 2003).

Physician/HCP Involvement

Briss and colleagues' (2004) initial discussion of shared and informed decision making referred primarily to patient–provider communication. These authors advocate population-based interventions to facilitate informed decision making (IDM) prior to patient–provider treatment discussions. Specifically, they conducted a systematic review of preventive cancer screening interventions and developed a model for IDM. This model includes patient and community interventions, focus on assessment of knowledge and health literacy, and discussion of decisional conflict or uncertainties. Briss and colleagues (2004) stated that more information is needed regarding individuals' desire for involvement in medical decision making, how to promote decisions that are consistent with individuals' values, how to conduct effective and cost-effective community interventions to promote informed decision making, and how to promote cultural competence in fitting community interventions to diverse populations. These issues are directly applicable to end-of-life treatment discussions and completion of advance directives; hence, it is important for clinicians facilitating such discussions to recognize these issues. However, it is also important for clinicians to remember that such discussions are not currently reimbursable (Tinetti, 2012), and, therefore, the motivation of HCPs to engage in such discussions with their patients might be low. Consequently, clinicians might want to focus on shared decision making between individuals and members of their social support network, such as family and friends rather than attempting to intervene as part of an interprofessional treatment team in patient–HCP decision making.

Family Involvement and Racial Differences

Decisions regarding advance care planning rarely happen in isolation. Family members of the dying person are often involved, whether in a formal process (i.e., as a partner in creating an advance directive) or an informal one (i.e., conversations about preferences). In a sample of adults aged 64 to 65, 75% reported having informal conversations, the vast majority of these with family members (Carr & Khodyakov, 2007). Family involvement during end-of-life decision making is common and may systematically contribute to the specific treatment decisions being made. Simply having informal conversations with loved ones about treatment preferences has been found to be a robust predictor of the likelihood that one has formal plans (Carr & Khodyakov, 2007).

For example, patients who died in a hospital with family present were more likely to have a DNR order (e.g., a formal plan and a type of advance directive), to withdraw treatments in the last 2 days of life, and to receive narcotics consistent with comfort care (Tschann et al., 2003). The level of family involvement and influence in advance care planning, however, may vary among different cultures (Bullock, 2011). For ethnic minorities, family support, and inclusion has been consistent in the literature, such as among Hispanics and African Americans where, culturally, the use of family to communicate the wishes of the patient is often seen as more relevant to the medical situation than a written directive (Volker, 2005). Perkins and colleagues (2002) concluded that among Mexican Americans, the health care system and family both were trusted to serve the patient's interest in a study about cross-cultural similarities and differences in attitudes about advance care planning. In the same study, African Americans disclosed their wishes to their family but were less likely to discuss treatment wishes with their HCP. The authors suggested that "trust" of the health care system was a potential factor in this difference. African Americans believe that the health care system controls treatment and they lack trust in this system to serve them well (Crawley et al., 2000; Krakauer et al., 2002).

African Americans, however, trust their families to promote their wishes regarding advance directives and end-of-life care. Schmid and colleagues (2010) found higher treatment preference agreement among African American dyads compared to Caucasian dyads consisting primarily of older adults and their adult children. Prior advance care planning moderated the effect, such that African American and Caucasian dyads did not differ in treatment preference agreement at high levels of advance care planning. At lower levels of advance care planning, however, African American proxies made undertreatment errors, whereas Caucasian proxies made overtreatment errors. As clinicians, facilitating and tailoring the approach to conversations about advance directives may help to remove obstacles and address any misconceptions among the individual or family members involved.

CASE 1: ELDER LAW CLINIC GEROPSYCHOLOGY CONSULTATION AND DECISIONAL CAPACITY

Mrs. Harris and her two adult daughters, all self-identifying as African American, were referred by their attorney to the Elder Law Clinic Geropsychology Consultation Service. The attorney was uncertain as to Mrs. Harris's capacity to designate a specific proxy (i.e., one of her adult daughters) as durable power of attorney and power of attorney for health care. Depending on the state, a durable power of attorney typically covers financial matters after the individual in question has become unable to direct his or her own finances or communicate his or her financial wishes. In contrast, a durable power of attorney for health care designates a specific proxy to make health care decisions on a person's behalf if he or she becomes unable to do so (Alzheimer's Association, 2011).

Mrs. Harris, an 83-year-old retired domestic worker who had completed 10th grade, had been living for the past 3 years with her daughter Anne. Mrs. Harris's other daughter, Peggy, visited at least four times per week and provided respite services, or took Mrs. Harris into her own home when Anne needed to travel or attend to other family tasks for her three children.

Mrs. Harris had been diagnosed with dementia 4 years previously by her family practice physician. This diagnosis was supported by Mrs. Harris's low score in the education-adjusted dementia range on a brief cognitive screening measure. The low score did not seem to be influenced by any depressive symptoms, as Mrs. Harris's score on a brief depression scale was quite low. The clinical assessment revealed that Mrs. Harris clearly had a diminished working memory capacity and a compromised ability to express herself in a rational and eloquent manner. This deficiency was especially poignant when she was asked to remember, process, and respond to newly presented information.

Based on a standardized capacity assessment interview, however, Mrs. Harris did seem to maintain the ability to comprehend and assimilate information if it was presented one "fact" at a time. She was also able to respond to simple questions about newly presented information when the questions were phrased in a manner that she could answer in a simple form (i.e., yes or no). Mrs. Harris consistently stated that she wanted her daughter Anne to make decisions for her, stating, "We are of one accord."

CAPACITY EVALUATIONS AND UNDUE INFLUENCE

As illustrated in the case above, it is imperative for clinicians and HCPs to fully understand the tension between individual consent capacity in the completion of advance directives and the need or desire for family involvement on the part of any individual, and to assess any potential for undue influence (Allen & Shuster, 2002; American Bar Association and American Psychological Association [ABA/APA], 2008; King, Kim, & Conwell, 2000). Any type of informed consent, such as that for end-of-life medical treatments or completion of advance directives, must be given voluntarily, knowingly, and competently. The case of Mrs. Harris illustrates a situation in which a supportive family environment surrounds an individual with compromised decision-making capacity. Sadly, not all family situations are supportive, and not all individuals with compromised decision-making capacity have relatives or other support systems; these individuals become particularly vulnerable to financial predators. Allen and Shuster (2002) discussed systems-level capacity and individual informed consent, including ways in which the determination of voluntariness, adequate knowledge, and competence or capacity may be compromised by family dynamics within the context of end-of-life medical treatment planning.

In 2008, the American Bar Association and the American Psychological Association partnered to publish guidelines for psychologists working with older adults with diminished capacity. One issue covered in these guidelines is "undue influence." The legal definition of undue influence varies by state but the overriding principle is the intentional use of social influence, deception, and manipulation to gain control of the decision making of another person (ABA/APA, 2008, p. 15). Hence, undue influence may exist in relationships based on trust and confidence, as would be the case among family members or friends. Cases of undue influence typically involve financial matters or creation of estate wills (ABA/APA, 2008). Cognitively impaired individuals may be particularly vulnerable to undue influence, but cognitive impairment is not a prerequisite. Although medical treatment decisions and end-of-life planning are not typically discussed in relation to undue influence, clinicians should recognize this issue and be careful in their evaluation of family pressures on individuals near the end of life (Allen & Shuster, 2002).

ADVANCE DIRECTIVES AND MENTAL HEALTH

Cognitive impairment and consent capacity are not the only mental health issues that clinicians may wish to consider when assisting individuals in the advance care planning process. Research has found a link between avoidance of planning for end-of-life treatment and higher depression symptom severity (Blank et al., 2001; Sörensen et al., 2011). Moreover, depression may reduce an individual's desire or ability to seek information regarding end-of-life treatment options (Sörensen et al., 2008). These results suggest that clinicians should be particularly mindful of individuals facing the end-of-life planning process while suffering depression or depression symptoms. This population may require additional support or concurrent treatment of depression to navigate the process of planning end-of-life medical treatment and executing advance directives.

Rather than focusing on the influence of depression on advance care planning and the completion of advance directives, Ganzini and colleagues (2010) examined end-of-life care for veterans with schizophrenia and those without major mental illness, theorizing that individuals with schizophrenia would have less access to quality end-of-life care. They found 63% of individuals with schizophrenia had physician orders to forego CPR. In contrast with a priori hypotheses, veterans with schizophrenia received comparable or better end-of-life care on most measures relative to veterans without mental illness.

In contrast, Cai, Cram, and Li (2011) examined the rates of four advance care plans among nursing home residents with and without serious mental illness: DNRs, living wills, do-not-hospitalize orders, and orders restricting feeding tubes. Nursing home residents with severe mental illness had a 24% reduced likelihood of having any of the four advance care plans when adjusting for individual and facility characteristics. These authors called for greater research examining individual characteristics and psychosocial variables as they relate to advance directives among those with and without severe mental illness. Moreover, it is imperative for clinicians working with clients with severe mental illness to be mindful of both diminished capacity and impoverished social support systems. These individuals are particularly vulnerable to undue influence and health care disparities between stated treatment preference and actual medical care at the end of life, as illustrated in the case example below.

CASE 2: GERIATRICS CLINIC CLIENT WITH MENTAL ILLNESS

Ms. Douglas, an 86-year-old Caucasian woman, was brought to the Geriatrics Clinic for evaluation by law enforcement officers at the County Jail. She had been incarcerated for 2 days prior to her appointment for trespassing and panhandling at a local fast food restaurant after her recreational vehicle was impounded and her four dogs were taken to the local animal shelter.

There were very few records available for Ms. Douglas; she had friends in the clergy in town but had no living relatives. She had lived a nomadic existence most of her adult life, picking up odd jobs to support her and her dogs during her travels. She had never applied for Medicare/Medicaid and, basically "lived off of the grid."

Full interprofessional assessment revealed a malignant neoplasm in her left breast, no medical indication of delirium, mild cognitive impairment, and a presumptive diagnosis of bipolar disorder or schizophrenia as indicated by press of speech, high energy, self-expressed need to finish her "Jesus Journey Journal," and potential delusions as indicated by her stated belief she was on a mission from God. Standardized capacity assessment revealed that Ms. Douglas did not retain capacity to live independently or execute medical decisions, such as choosing a specific treatment approach for her breast cancer. While social work attempted to find community placement for Ms. Douglas, she was returned to the local county jail.

ADVANCE DIRECTIVES IN LONG-TERM CARE

As stated previously, advance directives are more prevalent among individuals receiving any type of long-term care (Jones et al., 2011). Among residents of skilled nursing facilities, Levin and colleagues (1999) found that 74% of nursing home residents had a DNR order but only 32% had an additional written advance directive documented in the medical chart. Presence of a DNR order was associated with older age, longer length of stay, geographic location, physician–family member discussion, and the presence of an additional advance directive such as a living will in the medical chart. Teno and colleagues (2011) investigated whether skilled nursing facilities increasing the rate of DNR orders over time also decreased the prevalence of terminal hospitalizations in the last week of life. They found that facilities starting with low rates of DNR orders that increased their rates had fewer terminal hospital admissions than facilities with continuously low DNR usage.

Although prevalence rates of advance directives are higher in skilled nursing facilities, identifying residents in potential need of hospice care can still be difficult and problematic because of high rates of comorbidity and functional impairment among residents. Research has examined the behavioral characteristics of skilled nursing home facility residents within 6 months of death in comparison with similar residents who were not within 6 months of death. Allen, Burgio, Fisher, Hardin, and Shuster (2005) conducted a two-group secondary data analysis of prospective observational data from 10 nursing homes and compared the behavioral characteristics of 32 residents who died during a 6-month clinical trial to 32 matched residents who did not die during the trial. Residents were matched on gender and initial cognitive status. These authors found that residents who died displayed more verbal agitation, less time engaged in coherent verbal interaction with staff, and almost twice as much time restrained in bed in comparison with matched residents who did not die across the 6-month clinical trial. However, residents did not differ in typical markers used to identify nearness to death, including comorbid illness or functional impairment. They also did not differ in use of nonopioid or opioid analgesics. Clinicians working in long-term care, and particularly in skilled care facilities where the acuity level of illness is quite high, may wish to be mindful of these behavioral characteristics among residents in order to facilitate ongoing advance care planning with family members. Specifically, residents displaying these characteristics may require discussions with family members about terminal hospitalization and hospice services.

ADVANCE DIRECTIVES IN ACUTE CARE OR DURING THE LAST WEEKS OR DAYS OF LIFE

Research in ICUs has shown that DNR orders were associated with medical versus surgical admission (Cardenas-Turanzas et al., 2011), White race, older age, being unmarried, the presence of an adult child as a proxy decision maker, perceived inability to survive discharge from intensive care, and longer lengths of stay (Chang et al., 2010). Morrell and colleagues (2008) found that although advance directive status (i.e., having a living will or other legal document expressing life-sustaining treatment wishes in the medical chart) had no measureable impact on DNR orders, there were differences in DNR prevalence depending on whether a medical inpatient was admitted to a general medical unit or a surgical unit. DNRs were more frequent among patients on a medical service and occurred earlier in the hospital length of stay. Given that medical service patients were likely more able to have treatment preference discussions with HCPs than individuals admitted to the surgical unit, this finding makes sense.

In addition to cross-sectional findings regarding correlates of DNR orders, some research has examined changes in DNR execution across time. For example, Levin and colleagues (2008) found a 3% increase in DNR orders in medical records between 2000 and 2005 among inpatients at Memorial-Sloane Kettering. Adult inpatients signed 53% of DNRs and 34% were signed by proxies, with 13% resulting from physicians' orders. The median time between signing of DNR orders and patient death was zero days. In other words, even in acute care settings, completion of advance directives may be delayed until the very day of death.

The last-minute nature of the implementation of DNR orders is noteworthy. In Phase 1 of the SUPPORT Project (SUPPORT Principal Investigators, 1995), investigators reported that 46% of DNR orders were documented in the last 48 hours of life. More recently, Bailey and colleagues (2012) abstracted data on DNR orders in the last 7 days of life from the medical records of 1,069 veterans who died in one of six participating Veterans Affairs Medical Centers in 2005. They found that 63.7% of veterans had an active DNR order at time of death. Among these, records indicated that the order was written within the last 24 hours for 219 (32.2%), 1–2 days prior to death for 54 (7.9%), 3–7 days prior to death for 256 (37.6%), and more than 7 days prior to death for 152 (22.3%). Veterans with family members present at time of death and those who received pastoral care visits were more likely to have DNR orders. African American veterans and veterans who died unexpectedly were less likely to have DNR orders. Compared to those dying on a general medicine unit, veterans dying in the emergency department or an ICU and veterans dying during a procedure or in transit were less likely to have DNR orders. Mental health diagnoses were not associated with the presence of a DNR order in this sample. Clinicians working in acute care settings may assist individual patients and HCPs with the DNR process. Specifically, interventions that target ICU settings, facilitate transitions to less intensive locations of care, ensure the involvement and availability of pastoral care staff, and create environments that support the presence of family members may improve the DNR process in these settings.

Several studies have been conducted examining the efficacy of interventions targeted to increase the execution of advance directives and improve advance care planning among various populations. Although these studies have often yielded mixed results, it is important to examine them to understand the complex topic of end-of-life planning and better target intervention efforts. The next section provides a brief overview of several of these interventions.

INTERVENTIONS TO INCREASE ADVANCE CARE PLANNING AND EXECUTION OF ADVANCE DIRECTIVES

The Patient Self-Determination Act (PSDA; Omnibus Budget Reconciliation Act of 1990) constituted an important step forward in end-of-life care and patient autonomy, yet the impact on patients' decisions to execute advance directives has been equivocal. The Study to Understand Prognoses and Preferences for Outcomes and Risks of Treatment (SUPPORT Principal Investigators, 1995) was a 4-year research project that sought to examine the effectiveness of advance directives among hospitalized patients. The research team studied patients 2 years before and 2 years following the PSDA's implementation, as well as a third group of patients who received a randomized, controlled trial of the SUPPORT intervention aimed to help improve end-of-life decision making. The SUPPORT intervention, utilizing a nurse as a discussion facilitator, encouraged communication among patients, families, and physicians about treatment preferences. Ultimately, the SUPPORT intervention encouraged patients to complete an advance directive. Despite intervention and policy focus on increasing execution of advance directives, results of SUPPORT indicated that, among the patient groups, there was no difference in rates of recorded, formal discussions pertaining to treatment preferences, DNR orders, or attempted resuscitations at the end-of-life. In fact, the only meaningful change following the PSDA was an increase (from 6% to 35%) in proper documentation of already existing advance directives.

In 2001, Ditto and colleagues published results of the Advance Directives, Values Assessment, and Communication Enhancement (ADVANCE) Project, which examined whether instructional advance directives paired with informal discussion increased the accuracy of proxy end-of-life decision making. Participants were randomized into four groups where some were instructed to complete one of two types of advance directive either with or without an accompanying discussion with their proxy (e.g., directive + discussion; directive only; discussion only; neither directive nor discussion). Across groups, the intervention did not improve accuracy of proxy decision making. In other words, whether the proxy had access to a completed advance directive or had a conversation with the "patient" about his or her treatment wishes, proxy–patient treatment preference agreement was poor. The analyses revealed that proxy predictions of patient preferences were correct, on average, less than 70% of the time for potential future illness scenarios (i.e., Alzheimer's disease, cancer with pain, emphysema). In the cases where surrogates made mistakes, they tended to overtreat their loved one (ratio of 2:1 to 3:1).

Yet, although the ADVANCE intervention did not increase accuracy in end-of-life proxy decision making, both patients and proxies reported higher levels of positive emotions regarding the ability of the proxy to make treatment decisions for the patient (Ditto et al., 2001). Specifically, proxies reported more understanding, confidence, and a stronger belief in the importance of advance planning, while patients reported a small but significant increase in their rating of how well they believed their proxy understood their wishes and their perceived comfort with the decision-making process. It is possible that the scenarios presented in ADVANCE were too vague or generic to act as a learning tool for participant pairs. Clinicians should be mindful of individual patient and family or proxy understanding of treatment options and appreciation of the consequences of potential decisions made. Education of individuals and their support systems regarding these issues is necessary.

Indeed, Briggs and colleagues (2004) reported on a successful education-based patient-centered advance care planning approach (Pc-ACP). By educating potential patients and family members about the progression of the patient's medical condition, potential complications, and benefits and burdens of available treatments, this intervention improved patient–proxy treatment preference agreement. The intervention entails a one-time, 1-hour interview with the goal of increasing dyadic congruence, advance care planning knowledge, and decreasing decisional conflict. The success of the intervention was attributed to the use of scenarios that were realistic and relevant to the individuals in question, as well as to the involvement of the proxy throughout the intervention. This study is encouraging for multiple reasons. The intervention employed was brief: a one-time, 1-hour interview, and was able to show significant improvement in concordance. Furthermore, the Pc-ACP intervention demonstrates that end-of-life discussions can occur in ways that reduce decisional conflict and stress, which counters the belief that engaging in conversations about dying is an emotionally or psychologically harmful process.

A more recent intervention targeted African Americans with end-stage renal disease and their chosen family proxy: the Sharing Patients' Illness Representations to Increase Trust (SPIRIT) project (Song et al., 2009). This 1-hour, nurse-facilitated intervention was able to show increased patient-proxy treatment congruence in end-of-life decision making by using scenarios that were specific to the disease trajectory of the patient with end-stage renal disease. The intervention also incorporated a discussion of spirituality and values in the internal representations both the patient and the proxy had about the illness. SPIRIT succeeded in increasing dyadic treatment preference congruence while simultaneously increasing proxy confidence in their decision-making abilities. Furthermore, the intervention was well-received and valued by the participants. Clinicians working with individuals and families in planning for end-of-life medical treatments should be mindful of the success of the SPIRIT intervention and take a family-centered approach throughout the process to increase mutual understanding.

The results of these interventions highlight the need for clinicians working with individuals, families, and HCPs to do more than mention the option of advance directives to their clients and patients. Rather than "informing" patients of their right to receive or refuse treatment by providing pamphlets and other informational brochures at the time of admission for medical care, advance care planning and the execution of advance directives must be seen as an ongoing, family-oriented process. Advance directives should follow the patient throughout the treatment experience, but during medical crises these documents may be forgotten by the patient and his or her family as attention is focused on the resolution of the medical condition necessitating treatment in the first place. Clinicians working in health care settings should be mindful of the need to educate admissions personnel regarding the characteristics of individuals who are more likely to possess advance directives to increase the effectiveness of information transfer.

CONCLUSION

This chapter has provided clinicians working with individuals near the end of life with information regarding the characteristics associated with advance directive execution, issues involved in shared decision making between individuals and HCPs as well as between individuals and family advocates, racial/ethnic differences and disparities in advance care planning and the execution of advance directives, and the importance of the environmental context of end-of-life treatment decisions (i.e., community, long-term care, acute, and critical care). Moreover, interventions to improve the ongoing process of advance care planning and the execution of advance directives were described. Two case studies focused on decisional capacity to execute advance directives and the impact of mental illness on treatment decision making.

One issue that requires greater clinical and scientific attention involves health literacy and the need for effective and culturally sensitive patient-centered education about advance directives and end-of-life treatment issues. It is plausible that patient-centered educational interventions such as Pc-ACP or SPIRIT may improve the individual's and family member's health literacy regarding the specific illness situation at hand (Briggs et al., 2004; Song et al., 2009; Volandes et al., 2008). Decision aids must be designed and tailored to specific populations in need of increased health literacy. Typically, decision aids provide facts about the illness, treatment options, and probabilities of various outcomes with the goal of adding clarity regarding health consequences to assist patients in making decisions in line with their personal wishes and values (Allen et al., 2008; O'Connor et al., 2007). Data indicate decision aids are superior to information provided during usual care in improving knowledge and reducing decisional conflict (Allen; O'Connor et al.). However, it is imperative that clinicians choose decision aids that are appropriate for the specific cultural, environmental, and medical situation pertaining to the specific patient and his or her family, within the context of a particular health care team and organizational culture.

Another critical issue for clinicians and scientists interested in therapeutic interventions for individuals and their support systems engaged in advance care planning and the execution of advance directives involves situations in which discrepancy exists between the advance directive and either: (1) the treatment wishes of family members for their loved one (Vig, Sudore, Berg, Fromme, & Arnold, 2011), or (2) the treatment recommendations of the medical team (Robinson, 2010; Sulmasy, He, McAuley, & Ury, 2008). Vig and colleagues (2011) described and discussed the implications of a clinical scenario in which an 82-year-old widowed woman collapses in a local mall and experiences rapid, life-threatening health decline. Her only son and legal decision maker expresses to the treatment team that his mother would want to continue receiving medical treatment in spite of multiple systems failure. Then, the woman's sister arrives from out of town with the woman's previously executed advance directive requesting comfort care only—no life-sustaining, or life-prolonging, medical treatments.

The sister states that this advance directive was executed after both witnessed the suffering of their brother during treatment for metastatic lung cancer. Even after the HCPs discuss the woman's advance directive with her son, he does not perceive that his mother's situation is terminal (Vig et al.). Clearly, this situation is one in which psychosocial clinical intervention is absolutely necessary for the son, his aunt (the woman's sister), and, likely, the medical professionals at the center of this treatment controversy.

The situation described above is not uncommon in critical and acute care treatment settings and represents fertile ground for clinical and research attention. In such settings, the ability and willingness of the medical team to have DNR discussions with patients and families may be influenced by the perceived futility of life-prolonging care (Robinson, 2010; Sulmasy et al., 2008). This situation has been labeled one of "moral distress" for the HCPs involved (Robinson, 2010). Thus, physicians and nurses may need supportive interventions to share their experiences of moral distress. They may also benefit from educational interventions to facilitate DNR discussions with patients (if possible and feasible) and families. It is possible that patient-centered discussions on the illness representations the family and HCPs hold in a given situation (e.g., SPIRIT; Song et al., 2009) may improve family–HCP concordance and reduce moral distress associated with the discrepancy between medical opinion and patient/family desire for treatment.

REFERENCES

Allen, J. Y., Hilgeman, M. M., & Allen, R. S. (2011). Prospective end-of-life treatment decisions and perceived vulnerability: Future time left to live and memory self-efficacy. *Aging and Mental Health*, 15(1), 122–131. doi: 10.1080/13607863.2010.505229.

Allen, R. S., Allen, J. Y., Hilgeman, M. M., & DeCoster, J. (2008). End-of-life decision making, decisional conflict, and enhanced information: Race effects. *Journal of the American Geriatrics Society*, 56(10), 1904–1909.

Allen, R. S., Burgio, L. D., Fisher, S. E., Hardin, J. M., & Shuster, J. L. (2005). Behavioral characteristics of agitated nursing home residents with dementia at the end of life. *The Gerontologist*, 45, 661–666.

Allen, R. S., Haley, W. E., Roff, L. L., Schmid, B., & Bergman, E. J. (2006). Responding to the needs of caregivers near the end of life: Enhancing benefits and minimizing burdens. In J. L. Werth, Jr., & D. Blevins (Eds.), *Psychosocial issues near the end of life: A resource for professional care providers* (pp. 183–201). Washington, DC: American Psychological Association.

Allen, R. S., & Shuster, J. L. (2002). The role of proxies in treatment decisions: Evaluating functional capacity to consent to end-of-life treatments within a family context. *Behavioral Sciences and the Law*, 20, 235–252.

Alzheimer's Association. (2011). *End-of-life decisions*. Retrieved from http://www.alz.org/national/documents/brochure_endoflifedecisions.pdf

American Bar Association and American Psychological Association. (2008). *Assessment of older adults with diminished capacity: A handbook for psychologists*. Washington, DC: Authors.

Bailey, F. A., Allen, R. S., Williams, B. R., Goode, P. S., Granstaff, S., Redden, D. T. et al. (2012). Do-Not-Resuscitate orders in the last days of life. *Journal of Palliative Medicine, 15*(7), doi: 10.1089/jpm.2011.0321.

Bayer, W., Mallinger, J. B., Krishnan, A., & Shields, C. G. (2006). Attitudes toward life-sustaining interventions among ambulatory Black and White patients. *Ethnicity & Disease, 16*, 914–919.

Blank, K., Robinson, J., Doherty, E., Prigerson, H., Duffy, J., & Schwartz, H. I. (2001). Life-sustaining treatment and assisted death choices in depressed older patients. *Journal of the American Geriatrics Society, 49*, 153–161.

Boustani, M., Peterson, B., Hanson, L., Harris, R., & Lohr, K. N. (2003). Screening for dementia in primary care: A summary of the evidence for the U.S. Preventive Services Task Force. *Annals of Internal Medicine, 138*, 927–937.

Briggs, L. A., Kirchhoff, K. T., Hammes, B. J., Song, M. K., & Colvin, E. R. (2004). Patient-centered advance care planning in special patient populations: A pilot study. *Journal of Professional Nursing, 20*(1), 47–58.

Brink, P., Smith, T. F., & Kitson, M. (2008). Determinants of do-not-resuscitate orders in palliative home care. *Journal of Palliative Medicine, 11*, 226–232.

Briss, P., Rimer, B., Reilley, B., Coates, R. C., Lee, N. C., Mullen, P. et al. & Task Force on Community Preventive Services. (2004). Promoting informed decisions about cancer screening in communities and health care systems. *American Journal of Preventive Medicine, 26*(1), 67–80.

Bullock, K. (2011). The influence of culture on end-of-life decision making. *Journal of Social Work in End-of-Life & Palliative Care, 7*, 83–98.

Cai, X., Cram, P., & Li, Y. (2011). Origination of medical advance directives among nursing home residents with and without serious mental illness. *Psychiatric Services, 62*, 61–66.

Cardenas-Turanzas, M., Gaeta, S., Ashoori, A., Price, K. J., & Nates, J. L. (2011). Demographic and clinical determinants of having do not resuscitate orders in the intensive care unit of a comprehensive cancer center. *Journal of Palliative Medicine, 14*, 45–50.

Carr, D., & Khodyakov, D. (2007). End-of-life health care planning among young-old adults: An assessment of psychosocial influences. *Journal of Gerontology: Social Sciences, 62*, S135–S141.

Chang, Y., Huang, C. F., & Lin, C. C. (2010). Do-not-resuscitate orders for critically ill patients in intensive care. *Nursing Ethics, 17*, 445–455.

Chow, E., Harth, E. T., Hruby, G., Finkelstein, J., Wu, J., & Danjoux, C. (2011). How accurate are physicians' clinical predictions of survival and the available prognostic tools in estimating survival times in terminally ill cancer patients? A systematic review. *Clinical Oncology, 13*, 209–218.

Christakis, N. A., & Lamont, E. B. (2000). Extent and determinants of error in doctors' prognoses in terminally ill patients: Prospective cohort study. *British Medical Journal, 320*, 469–472.

Crawley, L., Payne, R., Bolden, J., Payne, T., Washington, P., & Williams, S. (2000). Palliative and end-of-life care in the African American. *Journal of the American Medical Association, 184*(19), 2518–2521.

Ditto, P. H., Danks, J. H., Smucker, W. D., Bookwala, J., Coppola, K. M., Dresser, R. et al. (2001). Advance directives as acts of communication: Randomized controlled trial. *Archives of Internal Medicine, 161*, 421–430.

Downar, J., Luk, T., Sibbald, R. W., Santini, T., Mikhael, J., Berman, H. et al. (2011). Why do patients agree to a "Do Not Resuscitate" or "Full Code" order? Perspectives of medical inpatients. *Journal of General Internal Medicine, 26*(6), 582–587.

Ganzini, L., Socherman, R., Duckert, J., & Shores, M. (2010). End-of-life care for veterans with schizophrenia and cancer. *Psychiatric Services, 61*, 725–728.

Guo, Y., Palmer, J. L., Bianti, J., Konzen, B., Shin, K., & Bruera, E. (2010). Advance directives and do-not-resuscitate orders in patients with cancer with metastatic spinal cord compression: Advanced care planning implications. *Journal of Palliative Medicine, 13*, 513–517.

Hanchate, A., Kronman, A. C., Young-Xu, Y., Ash, A. S., & Emanuel, E. (2009). Racial and ethnic differences in end-of-life costs: Why do minorities cost more than Whites? *Archives of Internal Medicine, 169*(5), 493–501.

Hopp, F. P., & Duffy, S. A. (2000). Racial variations in end-of-life care. *Journal of the American Geriatrics Society, 48*, 658–663.

Jones, A. L., Moss, A. J., & Harris-Kojetin, L. D. (2011). *Use of advance directives in long-term care populations.* Atlanta, GA: Center for Disease Control and Prevention, National Center for Health Statistics.

King, D. A., Kim, S. Y. H., & Conwell, Y. (2000). Family matters: A social systems perspective on physician-assisted suicide and the older adult. *Psychology, Public Policy, and Law, 6*, 434–451.

Krakauer, E. L., Crenner, C., & Fox, K. (2002). Barriers to optimum end-of-life care for minority patients. *Journal of the American Geriatrics Society, 50*, 182–190.

Kwak, J., & Haley, W. E. (2005). Current research findings on end-of-life decision making among racially or ethnically diverse groups. *The Gerontologist, 45*, 634–641. doi: 10.1093/geront/45.5.634.

Levin, J. R., Wenger, N. S., Ouslander, J. G., Zellman, G., Schnelle, J. F., Buchanan, J. L. et al. (1999). Life-sustaining treatment decisions for nursing home residents: Who discusses, who decides and what is decided? *Journal of the American Geriatrics Society, 47*, 82–87.

Levin, T. T., Li, Y., Weiner, J. S., Lewis, F., Bartell, A., Piercy, J. et al. (2008). How do-not-resuscitate orders are utilized in cancer patients: Timing relative to death and communication-training implications. *Palliative and Supportive Care, 6*(4), 341–348.

Moorman, S. M. (2011). Older adults' preferences for independent or delegated end-of-life medical decision making. *Journal of Aging and Health, 23*(1), 135–157.

Morrell, E. D., Brown, B. P., Qi, R., Drabiak, K., & Helft, P. R. (2008). The do-not-resuscitate order: Associations with advance directives, physician specialty and documentation of discussion 15 years after the Patient Self-Determination Act. *Journal of Medical Ethics, 34*(9), 642–647.

O'Connor, A. M., Wennberg, J. E., Legare, F., Llewellyn-Thomas, H. A., Moulton, B. W., Sepucha, K. R. et al. (2007). Toward the "tipping point": Decision aids and informed patient choice. *Health Affairs, 26*, 716–725.

Omnibus Budget Reconciliation Act of 1990, P. L. 101-508, §4206, and 4715, codified at 42 U.S.C. §§ 1395cc (a) (1) (q), 1395 mm (c) (8), 1395cc (f), 1396a (57), (58), 1396a (w).

Perkins, H. S., Geppert, C. M. A., Gonzales, A., Cortez, J. D., & Hazuda, H. P. (2002). Cross-cultural similarities and differences in attitudes about Advance Care Plans. *Journal of General Internal Medicine, 17*(1), 48–57.

Phipps, E., True, G., Harris, D., Chong, U., Tester, W., Chavin, S. I. et al. (2003). Approaching the end of life: Attitudes, preferences, and behaviors of African American and Caucasian patients and their family caregivers. *Journal of Clinical Oncology, 21*, 549–554.

Robinson, R. (2010). Registered nurses and moral distress. *Dimensions in Critical Care Nursing, 29*(5), 197–202.

Rosnick, C. B., & Reynolds, S. L. (2003). Thinking ahead: Factors associated with executing advance directives. *Journal of Aging and Health, 15*, 409–429.

Schmid, B., Allen, R. S., Haley, P. P., & DeCoster, J. (2010). Family matters: Dyadic agreement in end-of-life medical decision making. *The Gerontologist, 50*(2), 226–237.

Searight, H. R., & Gafford, J. (2005). Cultural diversity at the end of life: Issues and guidelines for family physicians. *American Family Physician, 71*, 515–522.

Silveira, M. J., Kim, S. Y. H., & Langa, K. (2010). Advance directives and outcomes of surrogate decision making before death. *New England Journal of Medicine, 362*, 1211–1218.

Smith, A., McCarthy, E., Paulk, E., Balboni, T., Maciejewski, P. K., Block, S. D. et al. (2008). Racial and ethnic differences in advance care planning among patients with cancer: Impact of terminal illness, acknowledgement, religiousness, and treatment preference. *Journal of Clinical Oncology, 26*(25), 4131–4137.

Song, M. K., Ward, S. E., Happ, M. B., Piraino, B., Donovan, H. S., Shields, A. M. et al. (2009). Randomized controlled trial of SPIRIT: An effective approach to preparing African American dialysis patients and families for end of life. *Research in Nursing and Health, 32*, 260–273.

Sörensen, S., Duberstein, P. R., Chapman, B., Lyness, J. M., & Pinquart, M. (2008). How are personality traits related to preparation for future care needs in older adults? *Journal of Gerontology Series B: Psychological Sciences and Social Sciences, 63*(6), P328–P336.

Sörensen, S., Mak, W., Chapman, B., Duberstein, P. R., & Lyness, J. M. (2011). The relationship of preparation for future care to depression and anxiety in older primary care patients at 2-year follow-up. *American Journal of Geriatric Psychiatry*, doi: 10.1097/JGP.0b013e31822ccd8c.

Stiel, S., Bertram, L., Neuhaus, S., Nauck, F., Ostgathe, E., Elsner, F. et al. (2009). Evaluation and comparison of two prognostic scores and the physician's estimate of survival in terminally ill patients. *Support Care Cancer, 18*, 43–49.

Sulmasy, D. P., He, M. K., McAuley, R., & Ury, W. K. (2008). Beliefs and attitudes of nurses and physicians about do not resuscitate orders and who should speak to patients and families about them. *Critical Care Medicine, 36*(6), 1817–1822.

SUPPORT Principal Investigators. (1995). A controlled trial to improve care for seriously ill hospitalized patients. The study to understand prognoses and preferences for outcome and risks of treatments (SUPPORT). *Journal of the American Medical Association, 274*, 1591–1598.

Teno, J. M., Gozalo, P., Mitchell, S. L., Bynum, J. P. W., Dosa, D., & Mor, V. (2011). Terminal hospitalizations of nursing home residents: Does facility increasing the rate of do not resuscitate orders reduce them? *Journal of Pain and Symptom Management, 41,* 1040–1047.

Tinetti, M. (2012). The retreat from advanced care planning. *Journal of the American Medical Association, 307*(9), 915–916.

Tschann, J. M., Kaufman, S. R., & Micco, G. P. (2003). Family involvement in end-of-life hospital care. *Journal of the American Geriatrics Society, 51,* 835–840.

United States Census Bureau. (2001). *U.S. Census, 2000.* Washington, DC: Author.

Vig, E. K., Sudore, R. L., Berg, K. M., Fromme, E. K., & Arnold, R. M. (2011). Responding to surrogate requests that seem inconsistent with a patient's living will. *Journal of Pain and Symptom Management, 42,* 777–782.

Volandes, A. E., Paasche-Orlow, M., Gillick, M. R., Cook, E. F., Shaykevich, S. S., Abbo, E. D. et al. (2008). Health literacy not race predicts end-of-life care preferences. *Journal of Palliative Medicine, 11*(5), 754–761.

Volker, D. L. (2005). Control and end-of-life care: Does ethnicity matter? *American Journal of Hospice and Palliative Medicine, 22*(6), 442–446.

4

Health Care Teams Working With People Near the End of Life

KIMBERLY HIROTO AND JULIA KASL-GODLEY

Mental health providers working with individuals with serious or terminal illness and their families find themselves interacting with an array of health care professionals and teams, given that the needs of these individuals often are extensive and can exhaust the expertise and training of any one discipline (Geriatrics Interdisciplinary Advisory Group, 2006; Hall, 2005). Although very rewarding, working on, or consulting with, health care teams can be challenging. This chapter will assist mental health providers in navigating health care teams, particularly those teams providing care to patients with serious or terminal illness and their families. First, we provide a brief definition of teams and a description of common types of health care teams, then we discuss elements of team organization and factors that can impinge on or facilitate team organization and, thus, the delivery of palliative and end-of-life care.

CASE 1:

Consider the case of Mr. Smith, a 60-year-old, European American man with a malignant, inoperable tumor along his spinal cord. Since developing the tumor 7 years ago he requires increasingly frequent periods of ventilator assistance. Mr. Smith now presents to an inpatient medical rehabilitation setting for a routine evaluation to assess physical and psychosocial functioning. Unfortunately, he experienced a precipitous decline, becoming ventilator dependent prompting his placement in a shared room for patients rehabilitating with ventilator assistance. He required a tracheostomy and the medical team determined that he would require ventilator assistance indefinitely despite their attempts to wean him off it. Mr. Smith reminisced about his formerly carefree lifestyle and his love for the aesthetics, including his hair, nonconformist fashion, and passion for traveling. He reflected on his process of adjusting to the effects of the tumor over these 7 years and contrasted his former lifestyle to his current one—paralyzed in a hospital bed with limited movement of his hands. He described the impact of having to wear the same, nondescript hospital pajamas, depend on others to eat and bathe, and the need to relinquish his jewelry, even though he fought to wear his earrings as a reminder of his autonomy and unique identity.

His wife, a 53-year-old first-generation African Caribbean American, educated herself about her husband's condition and needs and became a strong advocate for him. She served as his primary caregiver at home and worked hard to enhance his quality of life. However, despite her dedication, Mr. Smith reported a significant change in his quality of life. Although he adjusted as well as possible to these gradual changes to his way of life, on many occasions he expressed his decreased will to live. His wife struggled seeing her husband decline in both function and spirit, and although troubled by her own ambivalence about his life, continued encouraging him to "fight."

Over the course of several weeks and without improvement in functioning, Mr. Smith consistently endorsed his wish to forego monitoring of his general health status (e.g., stopping insulin injections, refraining from blood pressure checks) and opted instead for comfort measures. Mr. Smith's attending physician talked with the rehabilitation team, as well as Mr. Smith and his wife, about requesting a consultation from the palliative care consult team to facilitate goals of care conversations, assist with symptom management (such as physical pain, anxiety), and offer additional support to Mr. and Mrs. Smith. Mrs. Smith was angry about her husband's wishes and wanted him not to "give up." Although she recognized his perspective, she could not imagine life without her husband. The rehabilitation team also expressed their concerns, specifically about the amount of pain medications prescribed for Mr. Smith and about the trajectory of Mr. Smith's decline in the ventilator room and how his eventual dying process might affect the morale of other patients in this room who nearly died from their spinal cord injuries and were striving to recover. Ultimately, a referral to the palliative care consult team was made.

As one can see from this case, to which we will return, in addition to Mr. Smith and his wife, multiple providers are involved and hold differing views about how to best care for him.

HEALTH CARE TEAMS DEFINED

A team is a group of people possessing a particular expertise, who meet together to collaborate and coordinate information and activities in order to achieve a common goal. The goals for health care teams often are twofold: to direct patient care and to do "team work," that is, attending to the process of working together in addition to the quality and effectiveness of patient outcomes.

Several types of teams are common in health care (see Exhibit 4.1). In *multidisciplinary teams*, members of different disciplines work together but function independently, with minimal coordination or consultation with each other regarding care. Individual disciplines own their treatment plan, though they often integrate input from others. Multidisciplinary teams are hierarchically organized and leadership and decision making are not shared (Lickiss, Turner, & Pollock, 2004; Zeiss & Gallagher-Thompson, 2003; Zeiss & Steffen, 1996, 1998). Decision making is vertical—so even if collaborative, one person has the final say, which can result in team members feeling ineffectual or undervalued. However, decision making tends to be quick, which can be an advantage in times of crisis or when decisions are straightforward or do not require multiple perspectives (e.g., managing a patient's medical symptoms that do not have substantive psychological correlates).

Interdisciplinary teams are composed of providers from different disciplines who collaboratively and interdependently plan, implement, and evaluate outcomes of the care provided to patients and families. The division of tasks among team members is based more on patient problems and needs than on traditional role definitions (Zeiss & Gallagher-Thompson, 2003). Decision making and leadership are shared and flexible, and responsibility and power are equally distributed, when feasible (Zeiss & Steffen, 1996, 1998). Team members reach consensus regarding team goals and responsibilities, recognize their shared responsibility for patients, and acknowledge the unique competencies, contributions, and roles of each discipline, as well as the areas of overlapping function (Lickiss et al., 2004; Zeiss & Steffen, 1998). Although shared decision making is the ideal on interdisciplinary teams, it may be difficult to maintain equal contributions and responsibilities

EXHIBIT 4.1

Common Types of Health Care Teams

- Multidisciplinary: Clear distinctions between disciplines with little role overlap
- Interdisciplinary: Collaboration across disciplines, fluidity of leadership depending on context (e.g., palliative care consult teams)
- Transdisciplinary: Blurred roles and boundaries; tasks can be completed by multiple disciplines (e.g., bereavement phone calls)

across all disciplines. When no clear answer to complex problems exists, responsibility may be diffuse across all team members.

Although interdisciplinary teams may not arrive at decisions as quickly as multidisciplinary teams because of shared decision making, research suggests that interdisciplinary teams demonstrate greater overall effectiveness and efficiency compared to other types of teams (Zeiss & Gallagher-Thompson, 2003). Studies indicate that interdisciplinary teams are cost effective and result in improved patient functioning and decreased readmission rates to acute care hospitals, improved medication adherence, and better patient outcomes, particularly for older adults with complex health care needs (e.g., Geriatrics Interdisciplinary Advisory Group, 2006).

Transdisciplinary teams are comprised of professionals from different disciplines who teach, learn, and work together across traditional disciplinary or professional boundaries. Members are familiar with the concepts and approaches of colleagues from different disciplines as well as their own. Roles and responsibilities are shared, disciplinary lines are blurred, and there are few seams between the members' functions, often resulting in the phenomenon known as "role release" (Larson, 1993). Transdisciplinary teams may require more negotiation to decide which team member assumes responsibility for a task because the usual default option of "this is the social worker role (or psychologist role or nurse role)" is not invoked. These types of teams are less common, particularly when patients need the special skills of specific disciplines. More commonly, teams use a transdisciplinary approach to certain tasks and an interdisciplinary or even multidisciplinary approach for other tasks (e.g., administrative responsibilities).

TEAMS PROVIDING PALLIATIVE CARE

One of the most common types of health care teams following individuals with advanced and potentially terminal illnesses, particularly in hospital settings, is palliative care consult teams. These teams typically are composed of a physician, nurse/nurse practitioner, social worker, and chaplain (Billings & Pantilat, 2001), though the teams may be expanded to include a range of professionals. Palliative care consult teams assist the primary treatment team with goals of care discussions, treatment planning, symptom management, emotional and spiritual support, and communication among and between medically ill individuals, family members, and health care providers. The palliative care consult team also may help initiate referrals with community hospice or home care agencies, depending on treatment goals. Often, one of their primary tasks is to clarify misconceptions about the definition of palliative care and its relationship to hospice or end-of-life care.

"Palliative care" is a broad term that refers to care provided at any point in the trajectory of an illness with the defining characteristics being a focus on alleviating physical and psycho–social–spiritual suffering, enhancing quality of life, effectively managing symptoms, and offering comprehensive, interdisciplinary support to the patient and family throughout the course of illness, regardless of stage of disease (National Consensus Project for Quality Palliative Care, 2009; World Health Organization, 2007). Palliative care also helps patients and families make difficult medical decisions that enable them to work toward their goals, especially as outcomes become more uncertain. Palliative care ideally begins at the point of initial diagnosis of a serious, potentially life-limiting illness (i.e., illnesses that will cause, or substantially contribute to, a shortened lifespan) (Newby, 1996; Rolland, 1987), and can be delivered concurrently with other therapies that are intended to cure and/or prolong life. If disease-directed therapy stops working, palliative care can be the main focus of care. Although the primary focus is enhancing quality of life, palliative care also may positively influence the course of illness and even extend life if provided early enough and when delivered alongside the best possible disease-directed therapy (Temel et al., 2010).

Palliative care practice also encompasses care provided through the later stages of serious illness and dying. In these stages, palliative care includes "end-of-life care" that might involve referral to a formal hospice program, as well as support of the family through the bereavement period. Hospice refers to an aspect of palliative care devoted to alleviating symptoms and enhancing quality of life during the last 6 months of life for patients who accept that disease-directed therapy can no longer be of benefit to them. Hospice is often linked to the specific programs offered under the Medicare Hospice Benefit. Individuals receiving hospice typically must forego active disease-directed therapy, though interventions intended to maximize quality of life will be continued and even enhanced. In addition to meticulous symptom management and minimization of physical and psychosocial suffering, specific goals of hospice include self-determined life closure, safe and comfortable dying, and effective grieving (National Hospice Organization, Standards and Accreditation Committee, 1997). Palliative care and hospice emphasize the needs of both medically ill individuals and their families (National Hospice Organization, Standards and Accreditation Committee, 1997).

Palliative care can occur across the entire continuum of care, from the treatment-intensive hospital setting to assisted living or long-term care facilities, to ambulatory medical programs, telehealth and other outreach programs, and home care programs. Hospice services can be provided in the home, nursing homes, residential facilities, or on inpatient units. Although mental health providers working with individuals with advanced and potentially terminal illness may not find themselves as members of the palliative care consult team, they typically work in the aforementioned settings and are in a position to facilitate collaboration between the referring providers and the consult team.

TEAM ORGANIZATION

When working with palliative care patients and their families, it can be useful to consider the organization of the teams caring for them—the structure, context, process, and productivity of the respective teams (see Exhibit 4.2). Understanding these elements provides a framework for thinking about teams and can facilitate more effective collaboration within teams.

Structure refers to the ways in which a team defines itself (Cole, Waite, & Nichols, 2004; Heinemann & Zeiss, 2002). This includes the members of the team and their respective disciplines, roles, and responsibilities. Structure also refers to the development of the mission, goals, values, and norms of both the team and the larger organization, and the degree to which the team and larger organization work together. *Context* refers to the experience of being on the team (Heinemann & Zeiss, 2002), the overall "climate" of the team (Bower, Campbell, Bojke, & Sibbald, 2003) or sense of "team life" (D'Amour, Ferrada-Videla, Rodriguez, & Beaulieu, 2005), including the degree to which members show cohesion (e.g., coming together around shared values), pride in the team, and satisfying working relationships. Context also includes the degree of organizational support of the team, the types of organizational barriers that might prohibit further team development (or expansion), and the level of autonomy granted to the team. *Process* refers to the ways in which team members navigate stressful situations, negotiate responsibilities, collaborate across disciplines, learn from mistakes and prior experiences, integrate complex and new information received from multiple sources, and make decisions (Heinemann & Zeiss,

EXHIBIT 4.2

Team Organization

- Structure: Ways in which teams define themselves (disciplines, roles, team mission, values, goals at both team- and larger organizational-levels)
- Context: The experience of being on the team, degree of team cohesion, quality of working relationships, and overall satisfaction of being on the team
- Process: Ways in which the team navigates stressful situations, distributes responsibilities, and makes decisions
- Productivity: The team's ability to accomplish tasks and achieve goals

2002). *Productivity* generally refers to the team's ability to accomplish tasks and achieve goals (Heinemann & Zeiss, 2002; Langfred, 2007).

Multiple factors determine the structure, context, process, and productivity of teams, including the stages of team development, the type of health care setting and its resources, professional training models, and attitudes toward palliative care.

FACTORS AFFECTING TEAM ORGANIZATION

Team Development

Team development happens gradually and evolves through predictable stages, though health care teams can re-cycle back through stages, particularly with the entry and exit of providers, change in organizational policies or resources, or evolving team responsibilities. Tuckman (1965; see also Farrell, Schmitt, & Heinemann, 2001) identified four stages of team development (though not specific to health care teams): forming, storming, norming, and performing (see Exhibit 4.3). A fifth stage, adjourning, has been suggested (Tuckman & Jensen, 1977); this refers to the subsequent end of a team following project completion. Though health care teams may engage in discrete quality improvement or program evaluation projects, the focus in this chapter is on patient care. The following briefly outlines the four stages of development.

Forming
Forming refers to the initial development of the team and the normative processes of learning to work together to arrive at a consensus about the mission and procedures of, and/or members' roles on, the team (Farrell et al., 2001; Tuckman, 1965; Tuckman & Jensen, 1977). This initial stage often involves

---

EXHIBIT 4.3

Team Developmental Processes

- Forming: Initial team development, getting to know each other
- Storming: Address turf battles and conflict in an effort to develop team process and style of communication
- Norming: Attending to team process and communication to establish team culture
- Performing: Balancing team content with process, to work effectively and efficiently together

team members getting to know each other and their respective areas of expertise; clarifying their roles, and the goals and mission of the team; and identifying and reviewing information to facilitate team development (e.g., time and organization of team meetings, collective troubleshooting of unexpected barriers to decision making). Leadership typically is determined by academic degree (e.g., MD vs. RN), level of seniority in a given profession/organization (e.g., nurse manager of 25 years versus new physician fresh out of fellowship), or administrative role (e.g., medical director versus clinician). The structure of the team starts to emerge during the forming stage as the team identifies the disciplines needed and begins clarifying their team mission and goals as well as members' respective roles (Heinemann & Zeiss, 2002). These processes can lead to the next stage of development.

Storming
As the team moves through the normative stages of development, it enters the storming stage, aptly named to describe the level of tension and possible conflict among team members as they struggle to develop greater cohesion and functioning within the team (Farrell et al., 2001; Tuckman, 1965; Tuckman & Jensen, 1977). Members may resist ascribed leadership and challenge one another's authority as they continue to learn about one another and how to communicate across different disciplines and interpersonal styles. Although tenuous and frustrating at times, the process of storming reflects the team's need to find a common language in order to communicate effectively with each other, foster greater trust, and navigate conflict (Farrell et al., 2001; Tuckman, 1965). Team structure continues evolving during this stage, particularly as team members identify their respective roles and responsibilities (Heinemann & Zeiss, 2002). Team members' experiences throughout these developmental stages reflect their evolving team context, especially as team members learn to work together and navigate the larger organizational system.

Norming
With time, the team progresses to the norming stage in which team members develop norms for managing team tasks that align with their collective mission and goals. The team creates guidelines regarding the roles and responsibilities of respective team members and norms for team decision making (e.g., identifying who will discuss advance directives, conduct bereavement calls, run family meetings; determining the factors to address when considering admission of a new patient). The team eventually reaches consensus regarding roles and expectations that serve as important touchstones when facing emergent crises or conflicts. During this stage, the team develops a more streamlined structure. Team context typically improves as the team generates a smoother rhythm for working together, and the process of collaborating and cooperating becomes less effortful (Heinemann & Zeiss, 2002).

Performing

During the performing stage, the team functions effectively and efficiently, easily balances content (i.e., type of information discussed) with process (i.e., how this information is discussed), and handles tasks with greater ease by reflecting on and learning from past experiences. Team members demonstrate their commitment to the team and its mission by aligning themselves with the team (e.g., reflecting on systemic barriers to care rather than blaming specific persons), acting in accordance with their mission and values (e.g., focusing on quality of life), and considering the team's needs before their own, for example. Additionally, during the performing stage, team members model healthy conflict resolution and promote an atmosphere of trust and mutual respect for one another. Teams work their best during this stage, operating like a well-oiled machine rather than a collection of disparate parts. At this stage, the synergy among the structure, context, and process of teamwork positively effects productivity as demonstrated in patient care outcomes and team members' overall satisfaction with each other and the quality of their collaborative relationships.

Settings of Health Care Teams

This section describes characteristics of health care settings that can impact team organization (see Exhibit 4.4).

Organizational Policies

Mental health providers serving patients with advanced and potentially terminal illnesses may work in a variety of venues, including inpatient units, outpatient clinics, skilled nursing facilities, or client's homes. Policies governing the operation of the institution in which palliative care and hospice services are offered can affect team structure by dictating the scope of services provided as well as staffing, including the percent of full-time equivalent staff (e.g., full time, quarter time). Provider panels and schedules may determine which provider sees a patient and his or her family and when, as well as who can participate in care planning or family meetings. Moreover, providers' ability to see patients at specific times depends on the degree of flexibility each provider has to manage his or her own schedule. In some settings, policies may dictate caseload requirements, and when the caseload is large and consists of patients with high acuity of needs, providers may struggle to meet these bio-psycho-social-spiritual needs adequately. Thus, providers may have varying amounts of time to devote to direct clinical care, communication and coordination with other disciplines, or activities to foster team development.

Clarifying the effect of organizational policies on team structure and context can reduce miscommunication and perceived unmet expectations.

EXHIBIT 4.4

Settings of Health Care Teams

- Organizational policies
  - Attend to allocation of resources, funding streams, organizational policies and politics
- Differences in training models
  - Inquire about colleagues' training models and perspectives about patient care
  - Identify potential areas of discrepancy and overlap in training models
- Attitudes about palliative care
  - Listen for perceptions and/or beliefs about meaning of palliative care and find "teachable moments" to clarify misconceptions
  - Consider the personal meaning associated with dying and death among (referring) providers who may be less familiar with palliative care

For example, a medical fellow may express frustration that the medical social worker has not helped a patient find housing when such responsibilities are actually delegated to a different service line. Continuity and coordination of care may be difficult in some settings, especially those with limited staff, fewer resources, or high service demand. For example, a university hospital may establish a palliative care consult team by borrowing from existing oncology staff, but lacks the funds to support a dedicated social work position. The newly formed palliative care consult team social worker may not have protected time from her existing duties to adequately address consult needs and yet feels pressure from the hospital to meet all demands. Team structure and context may subsequently suffer because of unmet expectations and additional workload requirements as providers try to distribute traditional social work roles and responsibilities to each other and the medical social worker on the referring unit.

Training models

The providers' training model fosters their "professional socialization" into their discipline and frames the way they view and conceptualize patient issues (Clark, 1997). When the relative emphases of professionals' training models do not align with one another (e.g., the social worker's perspective of the family unit as the driving force maintaining a patient's distress compared to the nurse's focus on wound care to manage immediate pain), tensions can rise and conflict can ensue (Haley, Larson, Kasl-Godley, Neimeyer, & Kwilosz, 2003).

For example, although both medicine and mental health ultimately focus on maximizing a patient's quality of life, the medical model traditionally tends to emphasize an algorithmic approach focusing on diagnosis and treatment with less relative weight placed on the psychosocial–spiritual aspects of the illness experience (Mizrahi & Abramson, 2000; Zwarenstein & Bryant, 2000), though this emphasis is beginning to change, particularly within palliative care. In contrast, mental health (e.g., psychology, professional counseling) typically places greater relative weight on interpersonal functioning, systemic factors contributing to and impinging upon psychological difficulties, and general adjustment to problems in living. Social work traditionally integrates service access and utilization into their training model, although the relative emphasis of this model in practice may vary depending on specialization (e.g., medical social worker vs. licensed clinical social worker in private practice). Clinical psychology places particular emphasis on assessment and diagnosis of psychopathology and, like other specialties within mental health, designs interventions based on psychotherapeutic approaches and their respective evidence base. However, differences between training models' relative emphasis on aspects of human functioning (e.g., biological vs. psychological) can drive frustrations between disciplines, particularly if one discipline feels less valued or appreciated than another.

For example, when professionals misunderstand each other's qualifications and skill set and/or try to prescribe colleagues' professional responsibilities to specific boundaries, the team context (e.g., experience on the team), process (e.g., communication, navigating stressful situations), and productivity (e.g., coordinating patient care) often suffer (Heinemann & Zeiss, 2002). Mizrahi and Abramson (2000) studied the perceived quality of collaborative relationships between social workers and physicians. Although professionals from both disciplines reported adequate collaborative relationships, social workers reported less overall satisfaction than did physicians. Social workers reported needing to help broaden physicians' perceptions of their skill set and primary work responsibilities to include counseling in addition to assessing patients at admission and planning for their discharge. Providers' perceptions of being undervalued or restricted to prescribed roles can fuel interdisciplinary conflict and compromise the functioning of the team.

CASE 1: (*continued*)

Returning to the case of Mr. Smith, at points during the conversations with the palliative care team, admission to the inpatient hospice and palliative care unit was considered. On the hospice and palliative care unit, the core team of professionals, including social work, medicine, nursing, psychology, chaplaincy, occupational therapy, music/art therapy, and pharmacy, had years of experience working together, and a history of having trainees from multiple disciplines and at different levels of training rotate through this setting. Programmatically, the hospice and palliative care unit housed an interprofessional fellowship that facilitated communication and collaboration between disciplines. The nature of this training program and quality of relationship between faculty members fostered greater understanding and clarity around the differences and similarities between training models (e.g., chaplaincy, social work, medicine, psychology). Moreover, hospital leadership supported training within the unit (e.g., allowing the psychology fellow to shadow physicians, social workers, chaplains), which exposed trainees to different models of training and ways of conceptualizing patients (e.g., medical and mental health models).

Within this setting, the primary leader and timekeeper for meetings rotated by discipline each day of the week (e.g., on Wednesdays psychology takes this role), and team members supported this shared leadership. The daily team meeting had a set format including acknowledging patients who recently died and signing cards for their family members, identifying patients to be discussed, sharing announcements (e.g., a patient's or staff member's birthday), and checking-in informally with each other during or outside of the meeting. Additionally, every Thursday the team met to review care plans. The care-planning meeting began with a "reflection" (a transdisciplinary task spearheaded by chaplaincy) that allowed the team a moment to center themselves and reconnect (through laughter, music, art) before continuing with their meeting. Team members spoke openly and respectfully to each other, and tasks (e.g., family meetings) were initiated on an as-needed basis and by the team member(s) most involved in the case. Questions and comments by team members often crossed disciplinary roles with the shared understanding that statements and inquiries serve to improve patient care. Like many teams, the hospice and palliative care team had its frustrations and challenges, but the team context remained cohesive and supportive, and the team process involved reflecting on past challenges to learn from and better navigate current stressful situations.

In contrast, the medical rehabilitation unit on which Mr. Smith resided had a newly established team. Aside from a few providers, the majority of the team members had worked with each other for 1 year or less as a result of recent turnover in staff. This setting also allowed for training opportunities, but only within certain disciplines (e.g., psychology, chaplaincy) and unlike the hospice and palliative care unit, trainees had limited interaction with trainees from other disciplines. Weekly meetings involving psychology, social work, chaplaincy, and case managers (typically social workers or nurses) focused on patients' psychosocial issues with a specified timekeeper. Although team members agreed on this focus for the meeting, the decision-making process of identifying a timekeeper stirred underlying tension about who held such positions of "power." Designated leadership was not discussed explicitly, but implied by educational degree and level of seniority on the team, which seemed to highlight feelings of resentment about perceived hierarchies within the team and a sense of being devalued for not being a "doctor."

Some team members expressed their resentment of this perceived hierarchy through their language use (the social worker referring to psychologists' use of "psychobabble") or actions (e.g., announcing the cancellation of this meeting when the two established providers were absent). Other team members reflected a sense of role restriction and of being prohibited from applying the full extent of their training and experience. Statements and behaviors of other team members also suggested a sentiment of "I could do your job," and a decreased respect or appreciation for the different relative emphases in training models. These disciplinary splits compromised the sense of team cohesion (i.e., context) and perpetuated a sense of distrust among team members.

Historically, the team functioned smoothly, attended to patient care and team dynamics, and generated treatment recommendations from discussions of patients and providers' experiences with patients. However, changes to the core membership of the team coupled with the personalities of some new members and their resistance to discuss their experiences working together led to the team reverting from the performing stage back to the storming stage as team members struggled to establish a new team culture. The current team tried instituting a similar approach to team meetings as before, but certain members experienced this process as intrusive and explicitly and implicitly expressed their resistance to this approach (e.g., coming late to meetings or not showing up at all, doing other work during meetings). Team members tried to invite open feedback about their team dynamics, but the lack of trust among certain professionals hindered candid discussion. Additionally, some team members' "professional socialization" may not have included feedback about interpersonal style, making discussing such issues within a group setting understandably uncomfortable. Although some team members wished to recreate the norms that existed previously, the degree of resistance and lack of trust among some members prompted the team to decrease the frequency of team meetings from weekly to monthly. The content of the meetings remained solely around patient care with minimal disclosure of personal experiences. However, many team members remained hopeful that more time and experience together could help repair this fractured sense of team cohesion and facilitate positive team growth.

The case examples above highlight the importance of considering how organizational policies and exposure to different training models (e.g., supporting interprofessional training programs; fostering healthy interpersonal relationships) can impact team dynamics (i.e., how team structure, context, process, and productivity interact and manifest). Moreover, the history of the team and its members play a crucial role in developing trusting and collaborative working relationships. High rates of staff turnover can contribute to a sense of stagnation and frustration because the team might remain in a perpetual state of forming and storming with little opportunity for growth. The different team histories within the palliative care/hospice and rehabilitation units demonstrated the impact of staff turnover in developing a sense of team cohesion and trust.

Attitudes About Palliative Care
Entering different teams in various venues and acclimating to their distinct culture adds to the complexity of navigating health care teams. Care cultures may perceive themselves to hold diametrically opposed values, particularly with respect to palliative care. It behooves consulting palliative care providers to remain mindful of the culture and values of the referring provider/team and how the presence of palliative care may affect interactions within and between the teams. Perceptions and beliefs about palliative care can raise interpersonal and interprofessional tensions. For example, tensions can rise because of a mixture of misperceptions that palliative care means end-of-life care or giving up hope, personal and cultural beliefs about dying and death, and/or providers' wish to protect patients. Moreover, some providers may feel less equipped to discuss topics related to life-limiting illnesses or have concerns that their own loss experiences may surface. The relative salience of these issues may vary depending on the setting or referral source (e.g., intensive care unit vs. rehabilitation unit; geriatric oncology vs. internal medicine) and providers' level of knowledge about palliative and end-of-life care.

CASE 1: *(continued)*

Returning to the case of Mr. Smith, over the months following his admission to the medical rehabilitation unit, members from the rehabilitation and palliative care teams met to discuss Mr. Smith's care. They managed his pain, needing to rely increasingly on nonverbal signs because of Mr. Smith's compromised speech (e.g., clenched fists, moans) and addressed his anxiety through medication, massage, and therapy. They also discussed Mrs. Smith's discomfort with palliative care (e.g., her belief that not monitoring his health status could hasten his death), Mr. Smith's evolving medical needs (e.g., pain management, prevention of pressure ulcers), potential decisions still to be made (e.g., eventual ventilator withdrawal), and the couple's increasing anxiety about Mr. Smith's dying and eventual death. Ongoing discussions between teams elucidated inter-facility tensions between their respective cultures. Conversations with rehabilitation staff members highlighted misconceptions that palliative care meant "giving up hope" and allowed them to share concerns that Mr. Smith's declining status would scare other patients or visitors in the ventilator room and "take away" those patients' hopes of recovering. Both the rehabilitation and palliative care teams collaboratively tried clarifying whether staff concerns were based on evidence that Mr. Smith's decline adversely affected the morale of other patients or was more reflective of rehabilitation staff members' anxieties and fears about providing palliative and end-of-life care.

With time, Mr. Smith's mental status waxed and waned, prompting the team to transfer decision-making responsibilities to his durable power of attorney for health care, Mrs. Smith. Over time, and with the support of staff (whom she considered "family"), Mrs. Smith shared her worries about losing her husband and her role as caregiver/wife, and her fears about being alone. Staff members also confided in each other about their own anticipatory grief and their concerns regarding other patients (e.g., how the possible decision to withdraw Mr. Smith's ventilator and relocate him to a private room would affect other ventilator-dependent patients). These lingering concerns, along with the nursing staff's anxieties about caring for a dying patient prompted a meeting for staff facilitated by the palliative care consult team. The meeting focused on clarifying misconceptions about palliative care (e.g., that palliative care meant giving up hope), listening to and addressing the concerns of staff, and empowering them with knowledge about caring for their dying patient. The palliative care consult team remained highly attuned to the rehabilitation team's dedication to helping patients recover from near-death experiences (e.g., spinal cord injuries) and their understandable discomfort about easing a patient's transition to death.

The palliative care team attended to rehabilitation staff members' personal responses and adjustment to this case knowing of their close relationship with the Smiths and of the death of the attending physician's father a year earlier. The palliative care physician invited the attending physician to discuss how Mr. Smith's case reminded him of his own father's death. The two physicians discussed methods of coping with the emotional and personal impact of providing end-of-life care and ways of practicing self-compassion when cases hit close to home. The rehabilitation attending physician shared his avoidance of talking in depth with Mrs. Smith for fear that his own grief would surface. The palliative care physician offered ways of talking about this topic while maintaining some emotional distance and also offered to join the attending during these conversations. With time, the rehabilitation team members grew more understanding of end-of-life care and more aware of, and attuned to, their own and Mrs. Smith's grief processes. Several weeks later, Mr. Smith died peacefully. Mrs. Smith held a memorial service in the hospital chapel and created a photo collage of his life to honor the dignity and independence with which he lived and died.

The complexity of this case reflects the multiple challenges and rewards of working within teams in various health care venues. Mr. Smith's case elicited a range of responses and reactions from the rehabilitation team, including guilt and anger that they could not have anticipated and prevented his decline. The rehabilitation team members also demonstrated their wish to protect other patients' from seeing Mr. Smith's decline, possibly related to their focus on the survival and rehabilitation of patients who escaped near-death experiences. Although the medical rehabilitation and palliative care teams, in addition to Mr. and Mrs. Smith, appeared to have divergent goals, with time they recognized their shared goal to maximize Mr. Smith's quality of life to the greatest extent possible. Despite the common challenge of managing differences in team cultures and values, such as in this example, most teams find ways of working together to accomplish their goal and learn from their experiences to inform future development.

METHODS TO ENHANCE TEAM ORGANIZATION

Communication

Communication is the cornerstone of effective team functioning. We offer some general guidelines to consider when communicating with other providers irrespective of their permanence on the team (e.g., core member or consultant).

At a practical level, providers need to identify available spaces within their setting for meeting with patients or other care providers, determine their preferred mode for ongoing communication (e.g., text page, secure email, or voice mail), and clarify expectations about when and how often such communication will occur (e.g., scheduling a regular time to touch base, making arrangements to check voice mail during the day, or verifying that text pages have been seen and acknowledged for follow-up). Depending on resources, having a dedicated space for teams to meet, whether informally for lunch or celebrations or more formally for meetings, and having established methods of communication allow providers to share confidential or personal information in private settings. Well-performing teams remain fluid and flexible to the changing needs of patients, team members, or policies, and adjust their operations accordingly (e.g., moving a high fall-risk patient closer to the nurse's station for closer observation). Moreover, ensuring that providers have appropriate access to patient charts helps maximize information flow, minimize miscommunication, and decrease duplication of services. The frequency and pace of information-sharing also keeps providers aware of recent developments if they remain less readily accessible (e.g., remotely located) or only peripherally involved (e.g., consultants).

In terms of communication styles, mental health providers will want to share information in concise ways without jargon that clearly articulates the most important information and how it may impact other providers' roles and/or responsibilities (Kasl-Godley & Kwilosz, 2011). To increase the likelihood that other team members will listen and consider other providers' perspectives, it behooves professionals to convey their knowledge while still remaining tentative and open to questions and other opinions or impressions. Thoughtful, clarifying questions, rather than firm statements, often can facilitate this process. Using modifiers like "I'm wondering if ..." or "Is it possible that ..." can help convey tentativeness and still demonstrate knowledge and a framework for thinking about patient or team issues. Providers will want to be aware of their colleagues' training models, attitudes, and beliefs about mental health and/or about palliative and hospice care, and be able to clarify misconceptions and/or challenge stereotypes of palliative care and/or mental health care providers. Listening for the subtext within a conversation or the underlying emotions within a team meeting can help providers hypothesize about other issues undergirding the discussion (e.g., questioning another provider's judgment, feeling unsupported by team members). Tentatively raising these issues to the surface can facilitate clearer communication between providers and within the team and ideally foster even greater trust among colleagues. Of course, such discussions must be done with tact and great clarity in order not to compromise team context or process.

Conflict Management

Team productivity and thus, effective delivery of palliative and hospice care, depend on team members' ability to work through conflict and collaborate (see Exhibit 4.5). Conflict can result from a variety of factors such as personality clashes, large caseloads, deficiencies in communication, gatekeeping, clash of ideas, principles and values, poorly defined or disputed roles or role expectations (Lickiss et al., 2004; Oliver & Peck, 2006; Yeager, 2005), or unmet or inconsistent expectations (e.g., the social worker and psychologist do not know what to expect of each other) (Larson, 1993).

To minimize conflict with respect to the roles and expectations of multiple disciplines, it may be helpful to identify the functions each professional is expected to provide, based on the professionals' respective training and

EXHIBIT 4.5

Tips for Facilitating Conflict Management

- Identify the underlying issue driving conflict (e.g., differences in training models, discrepant cultural beliefs)
- Consider how the team has managed conflict in the past (e.g., do team members avoid conflict, discuss in private?)
- Consider if the current conflict reflects ongoing themes within the team that need to be addressed (e.g., perceived lack of respect for another discipline, strained interpersonal relationships)
- Remind team members of the team's mission and goals and find ways to remain focused on these goals in spite of differences.

specialized skills and knowledge, thereby defining unique skills and clarifying areas that can be a source of conflict because of role overlap. Mental health providers may want to detail clinical services that medically ill persons can receive from each discipline, deciding whether this delineation will be a generalized framework or specific to a particular patient/family situation. This process can be facilitated when providers take the time to ask about individual skill sets, as well as training models and professional culture.

Viewing conflict as the result of differences in training models and culture and recognizing its effect on team organization can help providers transcend their differences, see the complementary nature of their disciplines, and focus on areas of professional overlap (e.g., optimizing patients' quality of life). Moreover, recognizing colleagues' specialized knowledge based on educational background or training may provide clearer rationale for the distribution of responsibilities, especially if responsibilities are transdisciplinary in nature or not typically held by a certain discipline. This shift in focus also provides opportunities to examine patient issues from multiple perspectives, take a more holistic approach to care, and develop an even stronger "team life" that facilitates trust, respect, and clear communication. By doing so, team members enhance the overall organization of the team by addressing issues inherent to team structure (roles/responsibilities), context (experience of being on the team), process (communication, navigating pitfalls), and productivity (improving patient care).

Depending on their stage of team development, health care teams often have difficulty addressing issues of conflict, trust, and/or strained interpersonal relationships (Langfred, 2007). Honing skills and developing team norms for communicating and resolving conflict can help the team evolve along its developmental trajectory and enhance the context, process, and productivity of the team.

CASE 1: (continued)

For example, consider the palliative care and hospice unit that was being considered for Mr. Smith. At the same time, the team admitted a patient who identified as transgender and had only partially completed her transition from male to female. She was minimally responsive and although friends and some family referred to her as "Christina," her legal name remained male. Without the patient's explicitly stated preference to be called "Christina," some providers called her by her legal name with limited appreciation for how her name reflected her identity. Team members held off-line conversations to express their anger, sadness, and disappointment about the perceived cultural insensitivity of their colleagues and struggled to find ways of communicating their frustrations and emotional distress with the team. Members eventually brought the issue to a team meeting and collectively reviewed the hospice philosophy of respecting a patient's wishes and maximizing her quality of life. By returning focus to the team's shared mission, the team reunited around the common goal of placing the patient's wishes in the foreground and their personal beliefs in the background (Demiris, Washington, Oliver, & Wittenberg-Lyles, 2008; Reese & Sontag, 2001).

In contrast, the medical rehabilitation team, where Mr. Smith remained, addressed conflict off-line through private, individual conversations without addressing the issue with the entire team. During a meeting focused on patients' psychosocial issues, a team member jokingly shared a provocative comment reflecting her personal belief that living with physical disability was not a worthwhile life. Established team members met with this provider privately and discussed the insensitive and inappropriate nature of her comment and invited her to discuss how team members responded to her comment. However, she chose to forego this opportunity during subsequent meetings and neither her comment nor the overarching issues of respect and cultural sensitivity were discussed with the team. Avoiding discussion of the team member's comment reinforced the team's fragmented sense of trust and conveyed the message that the team could not and would not tolerate addressing conflict directly. Instead of closing the discussion, team members could have reviewed (or established) ground rules to foster respectful and sensitive communication without overtly calling attention to the specific team member. Like the palliative care and hospice team, reminding team members of their shared goals and values can facilitate team connection rather than condoning divisive and potentially caustic interactions.

Building Trust and Good Working Relationships

Several strategies can assist with relationship building, some of which occur formally and some informally. These processes occur over time and with conscious effort. Outlined here are some suggestions to help foster trusting and healthy working relationships. Incorporating meetings focused on patient care and team collaboration can invite team members to reflect thoughtfully on their experiences, celebrate successes, and learn from mistakes. Supporting these types of discussions also can facilitate greater trust within the team and demonstrate the value of teamwork in the service of patient care. In a similar fashion, identifying shared interests among team members regarding patient and family outcomes and care coordination highlights a sense of coming together over a shared philosophy and can raise providers' appreciation of one another's relative strengths and contributions on the team. Furthermore, conducting joint visits with a colleague from another discipline, when possible and clinically indicated, can increase providers' understanding of their respective interpersonal styles, training models, and approaches to patient care. Additionally, maintaining regular, informal, and brief communication with each other facilitates information flow and a greater sense of collaboration and teamwork.

At a more informal and interpersonal level, getting to know your colleagues personally and having candid discussions with each other also can facilitate good working relationships. For example, giving timely, frequent, concrete, nonjudgmental feedback about how a colleague's behavior affects you and why, conveys respect, trust, and a level of investment in your working relationship with him or her. The way in which you communicate this information ("when you said X, I felt Y") as well as your willingness to accept similar feedback remain important factors to consider. Being aware of your colleague's life beyond the work environment, including stressors in his or her personal life, also is important to consider as these factors may contribute to his or her current behavior. Offering to provide appropriate support in ways that feel helpful to your colleague and providing empathy as well as praise can go a long way in fostering greater trust between providers and a sense of interpersonal connection.

In a similar vein, celebrating one another, as well as personal events and professional accomplishments, frequently enhances the sense of "team life" and appreciation for one another and the team at large. Finally, breaking bread together, literally, often serves as a useful time to socialize, listen for patient or team issues, and get to know colleagues on a more personal level.

CONCLUSION

Some of these strategies require time that may not be compensated and is over and above direct clinical responsibilities, which can make it difficult to prioritize or schedule. However, time and effort devoted in the short term may be time well spent in the long term, if future challenges are avoided or overcome more easily. It can be helpful to consider what activities will build trust and support (e.g., meeting for lunch on a regular basis, organizing social activities for the team, or planning a retreat). Recognizing what works well and identifying opportunities for improvement and ways of negotiating disagreements also can help build trusting and healthy team relationships. Working together to improve team processes (e.g., initiating a Quality Improvement project) allows team members to join around a common cause, reflect on team dynamics, and promote a type of collective identity that often develops within teams.

Providers have multiple avenues for enhancing the organization and functioning of teams. Methods for improving team collaboration exist at the individual and team-level and vary in the amount of investment needed (e.g., having lunch with colleagues, establishing a dedicated space for meetings, creating ground rules for respectful communication). The importance of fostering healthy communication, conflict management, and trusting relationships reflect just a few of the factors to consider when trying to facilitate greater interdisciplinary collaboration.

Working on health care teams is complicated, at times frustrating, and incredibly rewarding work. Attending to complex interactions between people and disciplines and considering how these interactions affect team organization can be exhausting but worthwhile endeavors, especially when the team remains dedicated to improving its effectiveness. Moreover, enhancing the collaborative relationships between providers and fostering greater interpersonal relationships can make providing palliative and end-of-life care even more meaningful and fulfilling.

REFERENCES

Billings, J. A., & Pantilat, S. (2001). Survey of palliative care programs in the United States teaching hospitals. *Journal of Palliative Medicine, 4*(3), 309–314.

Bower, P., Campbell, S., Bojke, C., & Sibbald, B. (2003). Team structure, team climate and the quality of care in primary care: An observational study. *Quality and Safety in Health Care, 12*, 273–279.

Clark, P. G. (1997). Reflecting on reflection in interprofessional education: Implications for theory and practice. *Journal of Interprofessional Care, 23*(3), 213–223.

Cole, K. D., Waite, M. S., & Nichols, L. O. (2004). Organizational structure, team process, and future directions of interprofessional health care teams. *Gerontology & Geriatrics Education, 24*(2), 35–49.

D'Amour, D., Ferrada-Videla, M., Rodriguez, M., & Beaulieu, M. D. (2005). The conceptual basis for interprofessional collaboration: Core concepts and theoretical frameworks. *Journal of Interprofessional Care, Supplement, 1*, 116–131.

Demiris, G., Washington, K., Oliver, D. P., & Wittenberg-Lyles, E. (2008). A study of information flow in hospice interdisciplinary team meetings. *Journal of Interprofessional Care, 22*(6), 621–629.

Farrell, M. P., Schmitt, M. H., & Heinemann, G. D. (2001). Informal roles and the stages of interdisciplinary team development. *Journal of Interprofessional Care, 15*(3), 281–295.

Geriatrics Interdisciplinary Advisory Group (2006). Interdisciplinary care for older adults with complex needs: American Geriatrics Society position statement. *The Journal of the American Geriatrics Society, 54*(5), 849–852.

Haley, W. E., Larson, D. G., Kasl-Godley, J., Neimeyer, R. A., & Kwilosz, D. M. (2003). Roles for psychologists in end-of-life care: Emerging models of practice. *Professional Psychology: Research and Practice, 34*(6), 626–633.

Hall, P. (2005). Interprofessional teamwork: Professional cultures as barriers. *Journal of Interprofessional Care, Supplement, 1*, 188–196.

Heinemann, G. D., & Zeiss, A. M. (2002). *Team performance in health care: Assessment and development.* New York: Kluwer Academic/Plenum.

Kasl-Godley, J. E., & Kwilosz, D. (2011). Health care teams. In S. H. Qualls, & J. E. Kasl-Godley (Eds.), *End-of-life issues, grief, and bereavement: What clinicians need to know* (pp. 201–228). Hoboken, NJ: Wiley.

Langfred, C. W. (2007). The downside of self-management: A longitudinal study of the effects of conflict on trust, autonomy, and task interdependence in self-managing teams. *Academy of Management Journal, 50*(4), 885–900.

Larson, D. G. (1993). *The helper's journey: Working with people facing grief, loss, and life threatening illness.* Champaign, IL: Research Press.

Lickiss, J. N., Turner, K. S., & Pollock, M. L. (2004). The interdisciplinary team. In D. Doyle, G. Hanks, N. I. Cherny, & K. Calman (Eds.), *Oxford textbook of palliative medicine* (3rd ed., pp. 42–46). New York: Oxford University Press.

Mizrahi, T., & Abramson, J. S. (2000). Collaboration between social workers and physicians. *Social Work in Health Care, 31*(3), 1–24.

National Consensus Project for Quality Palliative Care. (2009). *Clinical practice guidelines for quality palliative care* (2nd ed.). Pittsburgh, PA: Author.

National Hospice Organization, Standards Accreditation Committee. (1997). *A pathway for patients and families facing terminal illness.* Alexandria, VA: Author.

Newby, N. M. (1996). Chronic illness and the family life-cycle. *Journal of Advanced Nursing, 23*, 786–791.

Oliver, D. P., & Peck, M. (2006). Inside the interdisciplinary team experiences of hospice workers. *Journal of Social Work in End-of-Life and Palliative Care, 2*(3), 7–21.

Reese, D. J., & Sontag, M. A. (2001). Successful interprofessional collaboration on the hospice team. *Health and Social Work, 26*(3), 167–175.

Rolland, J. S. (1987). Chronic illness and the life cycle: A conceptual framework. *Family Process, 26*(2), 203–221.

Temel, J. S., Greer, J. A., Muzikanski, A., Gallagher, E. R., Admane, S., Jackson, V. A. et al. (2010). Early palliative care for patients with metastatic non-small-cell lung cancer. *New England Journal of Medicine, 363*(8), 733–742.

Tuckman, B. W. (1965). Developmental sequence in small groups. *Psychological Bulletin, 63*(6), 384–399.

Tuckman, B. W., & Jensen, M. A. (1977). Stages of small-group development revisited. *Group & Organization Studies*, 2(4), 419–427.

World Health Organization. (2007). *Cancer control. Knowledge into action. WHO guide for effective programmes. Module 5: Palliative care.* Geneva, Switzerland: Author.

Yeager, S. (2005). Interdisciplinary collaboration: The heart and soul of health care. *Critical Care Nursing Clinics of North America*, 17(2), 143–148.

Zeiss, A. M., & Gallagher-Thompson, D. (2003). Providing interdisciplinary geriatric team care: What does it really take? *Clinical Psychology: Science and Practice*, 10(1), 115–119.

Zeiss, A. M., & Steffen, A. (1996). Interdisciplinary health care teams: The basic unit of geriatric care. In L. L. Carstensen, B. A. Edelstein, & L. Dornbrand (Eds.) *The practical handbook of clinical gerontology* (pp. 423–450). Thousand Oaks, CA: Sage.

Zeiss, A. M., & Steffen, A. (1998). Interdisciplinary health care teams in geriatrics: An international model. In A. S. Bellack, & M. Hersen (Eds.), *Comprehensive clinical psychology, Vol. 7: Clinical geropsychology* (pp. 551–570). London: Pergamon Press.

Zwarenstein, M., & Bryant, W. (2000). Interventions to promote collaboration between nurses and doctors. *Cochrane Database of Systematic Reviews, Issue 2. Art. No.: CD000072.*

II

Working With Clients Who Are Dying

5

Counseling Clients Who Are Near the End of Life

JAMES L. WERTH, JR.

Although counselors know that everyone will die, including their clients, many therapists may not be prepared the first time a client presents with a desire to talk about concerns related to a terminal diagnosis or if a current client receives a life-threatening diagnosis. Unless the counselor has training in topics such as physical health and illness, disability, the dying process, and grief, the therapist may not feel competent to provide adequate services to the client. Although this chapter alone is not sufficient to prepare a mental health professional to become competent in counseling clients who are near the end of life, it can provide an overview of key issues and some suggestions for further readings. Clearly, all the other chapters in this book are relevant to working with individuals who are dying, so the focus here will be on additional issues and resources.

The framework for the chapter is the set of "Issues to Consider When Exploring End-of-Life Decisions" that was developed by the American Psychological Association's (APA) Working Group on Assisted Suicide and End-of-Life Issues (Working Group, 2000, Appendix F; see also Werth, Gordon, & Johnson, 2002). Although the set of issues was originally developed to assist with reviewing end-of-life decisions (e.g., withholding or withdrawing life-sustaining treatment, who to name as a power of attorney for health care), the topics listed are also relevant when attempting to help alleviate a person's suffering or maximize the person's quality of life. Each of the major sections of the "Issues to Consider" is reviewed (see Table 5.1) and brief cases are used to highlight some of the topics reviewed. The cases are based on actual experiences but are combinations of people NS details have been altered to protect identities. The implications for counseling are highlighted, with reference to evidence-based interventions when such exist.

101

TABLE 5.1
Major Categories in the APA Working Group's "Issues to Consider"

Bio–Psycho–Socio–Spiritual Conditions
- Physical pain and suffering
- Comorbid psychological conditions
- Other psychological issues
- Fear of loss of control/loss of autonomy/loss of dignity
- Financial concerns
- Cultural factors
- Possible underlying issues
- Overall quality of life
- Other issues to explore

Social Support System
- Consideration of significant others
- Involvement of significant others
- Interviews with significant others

Systemic and Environmental Issues
- Indirect external coercion
- Direct external coercion

Note: From Working Group (2000, pp. 79–86).

PRELIMINARY CONSIDERATIONS

The "Issues to Consider" (Working Group, 2000) document begins with a set of five recommendations for consideration prior to becoming involved with dying clients. First, therapists need to examine their own attitudes, beliefs, and values and how these might affect their work with clients. If the counselor will be working in this area, then appropriate training is necessary. Further, it is recommended that the therapist finds an experienced consultant who can help with case review and discussion of whether personal values are interfering with client care and, therefore, referral is indicated. Collaboration with the health care team is also necessary. Finally, as is the case in any potentially controversial area, detailed case notes are necessary to explain why certain areas were explored and others were not.

CASE 1:

John is a Licensed Professional Counselor who has 10 years of experience working with clients who have traditional mental health issues such as depression and anxiety. Over the years, several clients have had health-related concerns but when one of his on-going clients, Mary, came to a session indicating that she had recently been in the hospital and was diagnosed with a form of cancer that could be life threatening, John realized that he was unsure how best to proceed with her. He also found that he was reluctant to talk with Mary about her fears of suffering a painful death, alone, and in the hospital. Upon discussing the case with a colleague, John came to realize that not only did Mary's fears mirror his own, he was being influenced by his own personal history. Both a paternal aunt and maternal uncle had died of different forms of cancer while John was an adolescent and both had suffered horribly. John realized that he needed to find someone with whom to consult about whether it was in Mary's best interest for him to continue to see her and, if so, how he could maximize his helpfulness and minimize the chances that his own fears would interfere with her care.

CLIENT'S CAPACITY TO MAKE DECISIONS

Although the client's ability to make decisions will not always be a matter of immediate concern, it is a bigger issue for individuals who are approaching death than for typical clients. Thus, the counselors will want to be able to make a quick initial determination of whether a more detailed evaluation is necessary. Beyond the issues of dementia or delirium, a person's ability to make decisions may be impaired by a variety of the conditions or situations outlined below. If the therapist has any reason to believe that the person's decision-making ability may be compromised, then a mental status evaluation is a good first step.

The next task is to determine if the person is able to perform the following tasks as they pertain to involvement in counseling and to her or his particular health care situation (Working Group, 2000, p. 81; see also Grisso & Appelbaum, 1998):

- Understand and remember information about the counseling process, including limits of confidentiality, and about her or his medical condition (e.g., diagnosis, prognosis, and treatment alternatives)
- "Appreciate the consequences (i.e., costs and benefits) of different possible decisions"
- "Demonstrate a clearly held and consistent underlying set of values that provide some guidance for making the decision"
- "Communicate the decision and explain the process used for making it"

The "Issues to Consider" document then recommends that the provider have the client sign releases to allow conversations and exchange of information with the health care team in order to help with treatment planning and clarification of discrepancies or lack of information.

There are some standardized instruments that can be used to help determine whether the person has the capacity to participate in discussions and to make decisions about health care issues. In particular, the MacArthur Competence Assessment Tool-Treatment (MacCAT-T)

(Grisso & Appelbaum, 1998) has been shown to differentiate among individuals with various health and mental health conditions whose ability to understand the issues is impaired.

CASE 2:

Rachel is an experienced counselor who has some experience working with clients around grief-related issues and related to health concerns. She recently attended a continuing education workshop on working with dying clients, primarily for her own benefit as her parents' health declined. She found the information useful when Thomas called and said he was referred by Dr. Jacobs, who said that Rachel would be able to help him deal with the news that he was in the early stages of Alzheimer's disease. Rachel decided to alter her regular informed consent process and instead of having Thomas read the material and sign it before coming in to meet with her, she reviewed it with Thomas in person. When they got to the end of the document, she asked him to explain it to her. When she was satisfied that he was able to understand and appreciate the issues associated with the form, he signed it and they began the session.

Rachel began by asking Thomas to explain what he understood about his condition and why Dr. Jacobs referred him to her. As they reviewed the information, Rachel started to wonder whether the mistakes she heard when Thomas explained his sense of what was happening were a result of poor communication between him and Dr. Jacobs, some cognitive impairment as a result of the Alzheimer's, a result of anxiety, or some other cause. She asked Thomas to sign a release for Dr. Jacobs and talked with Thomas about the possibility of him bringing his wife to their next session.

BIO-PSYCHO-SOCIO-SPIRITUAL ISSUES TO REVIEW

The set of "Issues to Consider" has nine areas to examine in this section, some of which are general and others have specific diagnostic conditions or areas that were identified in the literature. The first topic is *physical pain and suffering*. The primary concern is that many physicians do not have sufficient training in assessing and treating pain and other forms of physical suffering to be able to alleviate the symptoms (Lippe, Brock, David, Crossno, & Gitlow, 2010). Further, pain can make nonphysical symptoms worse and vice versa, so in order to effectively counsel people who are near the end of life, the therapist must thoroughly assess whether physical symptoms are being adequately addressed and perhaps act as an advocate for the client if suffering persists. Given the existence of palliative care specialists, no one should suffer from physical conditions, unless the person chooses not to take advantage of certain interventions (e.g., powerful pain medications) because of side effects (Graziottin, Gardner-Nix, Stumpf, & Berliner, 2011). Since most counselors are not competent to intervene to treat physical symptoms, collaborating with the health care team will be important in addressing the causes of physical suffering.

The second area to review is *comorbid psychological conditions* and the impact of these on the person's quality of life (see Table 5.2). The "Issues to

TABLE 5.2
Subcategories in the *Comorbid Psychological Conditions, Other Psychological Issues, and Possible Underlying Issues* Subsections

Comorbid Psychological Conditions
- Clinical depression and other mood disorders
- Clinical anxiety disorders (including acute stress disorder and PTSD)
- Early-stage dementia
- Fluctuating states of delirium and/or psychosis
- Personality
- Substance abuse (including accidental or purposeful abuse of/dependence on prescribed medication)

Other Psychological Issues
- Ambivalence or rigid thinking
- Fears (e.g., of pain, loss of mental status)
- History of actual and perceived trauma and loss (including traumatic head injury)
- Hopelessness and despair
- Internalization of societal rejection (e.g., self-hatred due to sexual orientation—"internalized homophobia"; internalized low sense of entitlement in women)
- Religious, spiritual, and existential beliefs, expectations, experiences, and values; sense of personal meaning and fulfillment in life; philosophy of life and life values; assumptive world components

Possible Underlying Issues
- Is the request for assistance in dying a form of communication and what is being communicated?
- Is there a "split in the experience of the self" such that the person wants the sick part of the self to die but the healthy part to live? If so, what impact is this having on the decision making?
- How is the person's ego functioning and related issues (e.g., coping and defense mechanisms, frustration tolerance, character scripts, locus of control and processing, cognitive style and biases, problem-solving skills, and ways of managing psychosocial transitions) affecting the decision?
- How are the person's specific strengths, skills, and assets, vulnerabilities, and liabilities influencing the decision-making process?
- Are rage, revenge, and helplessness involved in the process and what do they represent to the person?
- Are guilt, shame, self-punishment, and atonement affecting the quality of life and the end-of-life decision?
- Is the person viewing life as having already come to an end?

Note: From Working Group (2000, pp. 82–83).

Consider" document notes that these conditions may not make the person officially incompetent to make decisions but may impair decision making and therefore need to be aggressively addressed. Counselors will want to make sure that they are familiar with the literature on each of these conditions because they appear frequently enough that they will need to be addressed, if only to rule them out as areas to address in counseling.

The first and most frequently discussed topic is clinical depression and other mood disorders (Braun, Kunik, & Pham, 2008). The client may have had a history of depression prior to finding out about the illness or the depression could be reactive to the diagnosis. Determining the order of appearance can have clear treatment implications. The main things for the counselor to keep in mind are that clinical depression is not normal, even in the face of a terminal diagnosis, it is not to be expected or accepted, and it can be treated (Block, 2000). It may be normal for people to have symptoms of depression or of grief and loss, but these are very different from a full diagnosis of Major Depressive Disorder (Braun et al., 2008; Noorani & Montagnini, 2007). Treatment should be aggressive and multifaceted. Antidepressants may be useful, but if the person is severely depressed then they may take too long to take effect, so a psychostimulant may be in order to promote an immediate response (Orr & Taylor, 2007). The counseling approach will need to be determined based on the cause of the depression—there are evidence-based treatments for depression and these should be tried for the terminally ill person just as they would be for the non-ill client (Malhi et al., 2009). Given the fact that the person is approaching death, existential treatments may be appropriate and a combination approach may be the best.

There are two treatment approaches that have been developed specifically for terminally ill individuals and show promise through research. The first is Meaning-Centered Group Psychotherapy (MCGP) (Breitbart et al., 2010). Brietbart's group (2010, p. 21) reported that

> In response to the need for short-term interventions to address spiritual well-being, we developed MCGP to help patients with advanced cancer sustain or enhance a sense of meaning, peace, and purpose in their lives, even as they approach the end of life. (Results of a research study indicate that) MCGP appears to be a potentially beneficial intervention for patients' emotional and spiritual suffering at the end of life.

However, another study showed that the effects of an individualized version of MCGP (referred to as IMCP) did not have the same number and degree of long-lasting effects but there still appeared to be some benefits over a control condition of therapeutic massage (Breitbart et al., 2012). As a result, the authors concluded that the individual approach "has clear short-term benefits for spiritual suffering and quality of life in patients with advanced cancer. Clinicians working with patients who have advanced cancer should consider IMCP as an approach to enhance quality of life and spiritual well-being" (p. 1304).

The other approach that has received recognition in the end-of-life literature is dignity therapy. According to Chochinov and colleagues (2005, p. 5520; see also Chochinov et al., 2011), dignity therapy is designed to address psychosocial and existential distress among terminally ill patients. Dignity therapy invites patients to discuss issues that matter most or that they would most want remembered. Sessions are transcribed and edited, with a returned final version that they can bequeath to a friend or family member .... "Based on research results, dignity" therapy shows promise as a novel therapeutic intervention for suffering and distress at the end of life.

There has not been much literature on other mood disorders among people who are terminally ill. This may be because the likelihood of bipolar disorder being first diagnosed after a person has developed a terminal illness is small, given that most terminally ill individuals are older. Similarly, by definition, dysthymia must have predated a terminal illness diagnosis that was recently made because of the 2-year requirement for this condition. Thus, if either of these types of mood disorders are present for a terminally ill individual, the standard treatment should be begun as long as any medications (e.g., lithium) are discussed with the team treating the terminal condition.

The next major type of diagnosis of which to be aware is clinical anxiety disorders (Kolva, Rosenfeld, Pessin, Breitbart, & Brescia, 2011), including Acute Stress Disorder related to the actual diagnosis and perhaps Posttraumatic Stress Disorder (PTSD). Just as with the mood disorders, anxiety conditions could have predated the terminal diagnosis, so getting a good clinical history will be important. Some people who have had treatments previously, such as chemotherapy, may have PTSD as a result of their reactions to the prior treatment (Amir & Ramati, 2002). Similar to treating clinical depression, the interventions for anxiety conditions will probably incorporate evidence-based practices, such as cognitive behavioral therapy, along with some more focused attention on the terminal conditions. As above, MCGP (Breitbart et al., 2010), individual MCGP (Breitbart et al., 2012), or dignity therapy (Chochinov et al., 2005) may be appropriate.

The next condition listed in the "Issues to Consider" is early-stage dementia and then delirium and/or psychosis are specified. The primary issue here is proper differential diagnosis so that the proper counseling and medical intervention can be utilized. The literature is replete with reminders to not confuse depression and delirium and dementia because the treatments and courses of the conditions are clearly different (e.g., Dharia, Verilla, & Breden, 2011; Flood & Buckwalter, 2009a, b). One can certainly add psychosis to the list, because the hallucinations may overlap with the experience of people with delirium. The outlook for dementia may not be very good, even with treatment; however, if diagnosed correctly and early enough, the treatment for delirium may be as simple as hydration, attending to a urinary tract infection, and placing familiar objects in the hospital room or perhaps a short course of antipsychotics (Dharia et al., 2011; Flood & Buckwalter, 2009a, b).

Personality disorders are next on the list. The document notes that diagnosing a personality disorder may be useful to help the treatment team know how to work with the person rather than provide a focus for intervention. Several articles have been written for medical providers regarding Borderline Personality Disorder (e.g., Gutheil, 1985; Trimpey & Davidson, 1998). Similarly, it is not difficult to imagine how a client with narcissistic, histrionic, or antisocial tendencies could create chaos in a medical unit. Thus, therapists who are aware that these types of personality dynamics are present in their clients will want to prepare providers for the most productive ways to work with these individuals.

The final diagnosis mentioned is substance abuse, including abuse or dependence on prescribed medications such as pain medication. One of the problems that can arise when a person is suspected of, or accurately diagnosed with, a substance abuse disorder is that the medical teams may be hesitant to prescribe powerful narcotics because of fear that the person is faking the pain in order to get the medication (Ballantyne, 2007; Benyamin et al., 2008). Thus, it may be especially important when working with clients who have a history of actual or suspected abuse to involve palliative care specialists who are willing to prescribe medications to dying patients in the amounts necessary. The issue for the therapist may not be treating the person for the substance abuse but rather helping the person find the balance between dealing with the symptoms of the illness and maintaining lucidity to allow for interaction with loved ones.

CASE 3:

Robert knew that Stephanie had received chemotherapy for an earlier incidence of cancer but they had not talked about it in detail in therapy because that was many years ago and the focus now was on her recurrent bouts of major depression. They seemed to be making good progress using cognitive-behavioral therapy for the depression.
However, when she was diagnosed with cancer again, she spiraled back into a deep depression. When she said that she would "rather die" than subject herself to chemotherapy again even though her oncologist said that the cancer was likely treatable with a standard protocol of chemo, he thought that this was a result of the depression. Only when he took the time to more fully explore her experience of chemo the first time did he realize how traumatic that treatment was for her.

The third area to explore within the set of bio–psycho–socio–spiritual factors is *other psychological issues* (see Table 5.2). These are not formally diagnosable conditions but are related issues that could present in persons with terminal conditions and exacerbate the diagnoses mentioned above or could be exacerbated by a life-threatening illness. Instead of describing all of them, three will be highlighted here. Consider fears—not anxiety disorders but various types of fear—and how they may impact a person's quality of life, decisions, and interactions with the health care team and others. If a client has seen a partner, family member, or friend struggle with a condition such as dementia or suffer from unbearable pain, then witnessing and living through those experiences can lead the client to dread living through the same conditions. Fearing the same fate may lead the client to make any number of decisions that may appear irrational to an objective observer.

Two other issues that have been discussed in the end-of-life literature are hopelessness (Rosenfeld, Gibson, Kramer, & Breitbart, 2004; Rosenfeld et al., 2011) and despair (McClain, Rosenfeld, & Brietbart, 2003) or demoralization (Clarke, Kissane, Trauer, & Smith, 2005; Wein, Sulkes, & Stemmer, 2010). The connection between hopelessness and clinical depression is evident in the standard mental health literature and it is present in dying clients as well. Several studies have indicated that just as hopelessness is linked to suicidality in nonphysically ill individuals, it is associated with desire for hastened death among chronically and terminally ill individuals (e.g., Rosenfeld et al., 2006). In terms of treatment responses, it certainly would be inappropriate for the counselor to blithely reassure the client, but it also would not be in the client's best interest to accept the hopelessness. The therapist should become familiar with the literature on hope among terminally ill individuals and how it gets reframed from being hope for a cure to something similar to hope for a pain-free day or hope of seeing loved ones (Clayton et al., 2008; Johnson, 2007).

Another area that counselors will likely want to explore with terminally ill clients is "Religious, spiritual, and existential beliefs, expectations, experiences, and values; sense of personal meaning and fulfillment in life; philosophy of life and life values; assumptive world components" (Working Group, 2000, p. 82). The literature demonstrates how different *religious and spiritual belief systems* can influence attitudes and decisions; thus, therapists will want to talk with clients about how their faith may or may not influence them and whether they can obtain any social support from their faith families. Clearly, MCGP (Breitbart et al., 2010) or IMCP (Breitbart et al., 2012) could be useful in addressing these types of concerns, and dignity therapy (Chochinov et al., 2005) may also be beneficial.

CASE 4:

Sharon first saw Fred as a client when he was grieving over the death of his older brother from amyotrophic lateral sclerosis (ALS or Lou Gehrig's disease). Given that they had both been athletic through much of their lives, it was difficult for Fred to see his brother lose the ability to control his own body. When Fred, too, was diagnosed with ALS, he returned to counseling because his wife said he needed to deal with his fear of losing his ability to move. As the condition progressed, he became increasingly hopeless and although he originally said he would not kill himself because of his religious beliefs, when he was told by his physician that he would soon need to start using a wheelchair, he started talking openly about suicide.

The fourth area to explore is a specific set of fears that have been repeatedly identified in the literature as being related to why people say they want to hasten their deaths (Chapple, Ziebland, McPherson, & Herxheimer, 2006). Specifically, *fear of loss of control, or loss of autonomy, or loss of dignity* has been linked to requests for medication under the Oregon Death with Dignity Act (Ganzini, Goy, & Dobscha, 2008, 2009), which allow physicians to prescribe medicine to terminally ill patients who want to control the manner and timing of their own deaths. Given that these appear to be culturally bound beliefs, it is not surprising that the people using these laws are primarily European American, which is the ethnic group that seems to have the greatest concern about loss of control or autonomy. Thus, the obvious treatment implications are that counselors need to help clients determine how best to maintain or redevelop a sense of control over their own lives and futures. Similarly, if loss of dignity is the primary concern, then dignity therapy (Chochinov et al., 2005) may be the treatment of choice.

It is the author's own experience that many of his terminally ill clients would talk about suicide as a means of maintaining control. Thus, they would talk about their "right" to suicide if they were suffering too much. It was important to not overreact to these comments and instead see them as expressions of a desire to have a say in their lives. Many of them felt so out of control in every other facet of their existence that at least they could have a say in whether they continued to live. Once this was on the table as a coping mechanism, it could be addressed and agreements made for how counseling would proceed (see Werth, 1999). Of note, to my knowledge, none of these individuals actually ever attempted suicide but the thought that they could kill themselves if things seemed unbearable appeared to help them through difficult times.

CASE 5:

Carlos was referred to James by his HIV physician. James began his verbal informed consent process and Carlos soon said "stop." He stated that he thought he had the right to decide to kill himself if he did not think his life was worth living any longer. He said that if James was unwilling to accept this fact, then he needed to be referred to another provider. They negotiated a plan where Carlos would not take any action to hasten his own death without talking to James about it first so that James cold see if there was anything that could be done to help Carlos reduce or eliminate the symptoms that led him to believe that death was a better option than continued life. They were able to work together for several months on a variety of issues including depression, anxiety, and reconciliation with family. At termination, Carlos still believed he had the right to decide whether to live or die but also understood that he may not be able to clearly judge whether anything could be done to help him feel better, so he agreed to return to counseling if he felt suicidal in the future.

Financial concerns can be a significant source of stress for anyone but, given that over 60% of all bankruptcies in the United States are related to medical expenses (Himmelstein, Thorne, Warren, & Woolhandler, 2009), it is no wonder that people who are terminally ill often are concerned about the impact of their illness on their own and loved ones' lives (Emanuel, Fairclough, Slutsman, & Emanuel, 2000). Therefore, a counselor will want to make sure to thoroughly explore the impact that bills are having on the person's life and how these expenses are impacting the person's thinking and decision making.

CASE 6:

Paul and his family were barely making ends meet on his pay as a construction worker and his wife's income as a part-time teller at a grocery store. They did not have health insurance for themselves but their children were covered under a state program. When he was diagnosed with a medical condition that was treatable but would cost tens of thousands of dollars and would necessitate him quitting his job, they were at a loss as to what to do. Margaret was a counselor with a local agency that assisted people with little or no income. When Paul was referred to her by his physician's office, she worked with him and his wife to discuss options and identify ways that he could get the treatments paid for through compassionate care programs. However, even with all her efforts, the bills were still significant and the stress on the family was tremendous. Margaret continued to work with Paul and his wife on couples issues in order to help them maintain their marriage in the midst of the intense pressure that they were feeling.

The sixth area to explore is *cultural factors*. In addition to religious/spiritual beliefs noted earlier, other demographic characteristics such as ethnicity and age may affect a person's ways of thinking about his or her own dying. For people of many cultures, there is more of an emphasis on interdependence rather than independence, so involving loved ones in counseling may be important (Blackhall, Murphy, Frank, Michel, & Azen, 1995).

Depending on cultural belief systems, counseling may not be acceptable; so if a therapist is allowed into the situation, then it will be important to be respectful of the beliefs and values or the opportunity to help will disappear quickly. It is not possible to be familiar with all the different cultures, so therapists will need to be willing to go to the literature and consult with experts when working with people who have different backgrounds and belief systems from their own. For example, in some cultures, it is considered a violation of cultural values to talk in a negative way, so discussing living wills and durable powers of attorney for health care can be difficult with members of these groups (Carrese & Rhodes, 1995). The balance between respecting cultural beliefs and following ethical, legal, and regulatory mandates can sometimes be challenging, given the Eurocentric framework used in the United States.

CASE 7:

Sarah was a counselor at a university counseling center who was working with a first-generation college student of Asian descent who went by the name "Amy" at college but whose birth name was traditional for her country of origin. Aside from the regular struggles with college and not having much family support because no one in her home had experience with higher education in the United States, Amy was struggling with her mother's ailing health. She wanted her mother to go to a hospital but her older brother, who had the authority in the family, wanted to have her treated using traditional means and refused to allow Amy to take their mother to be treated with Western medicine. Sarah wanted to be respectful of the family's cultural beliefs and did not want to further alienate Amy from her family but also wondered what her responsibilities were under the state's elder abuse laws. She struggled with how to balance her alliance with Amy with her concern about the client's mother's treatment.

The next section, *possible underlying issues*, is a catch-all grouping (see Table 5.2). The "Issues to Consider" document indicates that "Resolution of the following issues, if present, should not be expected, nor required. These areas are listed because of their potential for decreasing quality of life and impacting relationships" (Working Group, 2000, p. 83). The items listed were taken from various articles in the literature or conceptual beliefs about people and their functioning. Thus, they may not all fit with a counselor's view of therapy or the world (e.g., some come from a psychodynamic perspective, see Muskin, 1998). However, therapists may want to use this as a reminder that there are theoretical orientation-specific areas that may be worth exploring, even if the evidence base related to terminally ill clients in particular does not yet exist.

Overall quality of life is the subsequent area to explore. Quality of life is a subjective determination, so counselors will probably take into account the types of issues reviewed above, as well as idiosyncratic matters of concern to the particular client at the particular time. Thus, if the client reports continued suffering even after the issues reviewed above have been covered, it behooves the therapist to delve deeper and consult with others to see what may have been missed. It may be appropriate or necessary to utilize some complementary therapies such as hypnosis, acupuncture, and "energy" therapy, depending on the person's belief system. The counselor must not be too provincial and limit treatment because, in the end, the bottom line is helping the person to have as good a death as possible, regardless of how that happens. It is up to the therapist to adapt to the needs of the dying person, not to force the terminally ill individual to die as the counselor wants her or him to die.

Finally, there are a few *other issues to explore* that are listed and are about end-of-life decision making (because that was the focus of the original document), such as history of suicidality, what end-of-life options have been considered, and what decisions have been made. These same issues are relevant to the counselor who is helping clients with broader end-of-life concerns and should have come up in the review of the preceding areas but, if not, deserve to be explored as well.

SOCIAL SUPPORT SYSTEM ISSUES TO REVIEW

The vast majority of people do not live in isolation. Thus, as has already been mentioned in the review of the previous material, it is very important to talk to the person who is dying about significant others and possibly involve those loved ones in the therapy process. As is the case with traditional therapy, unless it is an emergency situation, releases should be signed by the client before information is shared with any of the significant others.

The first area to explore with the dying person is her or his *consideration of significant others* and how the presence or absence of loved ones has affected the person. This first area involves looking at the degree to which the client has thought about the impact of her or his illness on other people and how the condition and decisions about the condition may impact significant others, including future generations (e.g., how will the client's death be explained to grandchildren who are too young to remember the person or were born after the client died). On the other hand, there are some people who may say that they have no one in their lives and the counselor will want to explore the extent to which this reflects objective reality (i.e., the person truly is alone, with absolutely no relatives or friends or anyone who cares about her or him) or subjective beliefs (e.g., the person is estranged from family of origin and friends because of substance abuse issues but there are relatives and former friends still alive). In either case, working with the person on altering the present situation may be worthwhile so that the person gets connected with a faith family or a 12-step group, or reconciliation is attempted with family and friends. Loneliness is associated with depression (Theeke, Goins, Moore, & Campbell, 2012) and suicidality (Stravynski & Boyer, 2001), so it needs to be taken seriously.

If the person does have loved ones, then an important issue to explore is the person's belief that she or he is a burden on these other people. Burden can be viewed in financial, physical, emotional, or other terms (Emanuel et al., 2000). Data repeatedly demonstrate that many terminally ill people believe they are a burden on others and that this affects their mental health and decisions. However, when loved ones are actually asked about their perceptions, many times they say that they get a sense of meaning out of helping the dying person (Enyert & Burman, 1999), which is one reason why the next steps, as outlined below, relate to actually talking with significant others instead of merely taking the client's perceptions as reality. In any event, the key to this first area is to determine to what extent the client has realistically thought about other people and discuss the impact these others have had on the client's mental health and decision making.

CASE 8:

Molly was estranged from her family as a result of years of substance abuse and related criminal activity. She has recently been diagnosed as being in her last few months of life as a result of advanced cirrhosis and hepatitis. She has been in and out of counseling and when she sees Jacob, who has been her counselor off-and-on over the course of many years, she seems different to him when she expresses regret over her past actions and when she says she does not want to die without making amends to her family. Given that she is in the controlled environment of the medical center and is too weak to leave on her own, they are able to make better progress than previously on addressing the mistakes she has made in the past and how she has hurt her family and friends. As a result of some active involvement by Jacob, Molly agrees to try to contact her siblings and ask for their forgiveness.

The next, and related, area is *involvement of significant others*. If the person does have important people in her or his life, then the next issue is whether the client is willing to try to involve them in their life and perhaps the counseling process at this point. Some people may have loved ones but may not be willing to tell them about the diagnosis or invite them into counseling. The counselor will want to explore the reasons for these decisions and evaluate the possible effects on the person's quality of life of the lack of disclosure or involvement. If the client does want to involve other people but has hesitated doing so to this point or is uncertain about whether and how much to involve others, then the counselor can help the dying person with taking the next step to increasing involvement, while respecting the client's concerns and limits.

If other people have been involved, then reviewing with the client what has happened and whether any additional discussions would be helpful and if the counselor's presence could be helpful would be another area to explore. For example, the possibility of miscommunication is high in the midst of such a stressful situation, so having joint counseling sessions with the ill individual and loved ones can help clear the air of any misunderstandings that may be interfering with optimal functioning as individuals or a group or may be influencing decisions by the dying person or any members of the support system. Finally, as the "Issues to Consider" document notes (Working Group, 2000, p. 85), "Review if there has been any direct or indirect, subtle or overt, actual or perceived, pressure from significant others on the decision-making process."

CASE 9:

There is an apocryphal story in the end-of-life arena regarding a family where Janet, as the eldest daughter, has asked her mother (Amanda) to come live with her and her husband (Steve) and high school-aged son (Robert) following the death of her father and because of Amanda's own health-related issues. Amanda reluctantly agrees but is concerned about being a burden on the family, a point with which the entire family strongly disagrees. A few months into the new living arrangement, Amanda's health has continued to worsen. After a series of discussions among Janet, Steve, and Robert, Janet sits down with her mother and tells her that the family has decided that they wanted to make a few changes. Janet says that they have decided that she would quit her job in order to spend more quality time with Amanda and help her around the home and take her to and from medical appointments. Because they will not have her income coming in, Steve is going to try to get some overtime at work and Robert is going to get a job instead of playing in his band and playing baseball for the high school. They have also decided that Robert will put off going to college for a while to be available to help out at home and by continuing to work and live at home.

A counselor who gets called in to see Amanda because her physician believes that she is exhibiting signs of depression and seems to be giving up on treatment may be quickly able to determine how miscommunication and misperceptions may lead to Amanda believing that she is a burden while the family believes that they are trying to show her how much she means to them and how much they love her. However, hearing only one side of the story may lead to the counselor not being able to effectively intervene.

The final section in the social support area is *interviews with significant others*. Following the signature of releases of information, the counselor can talk to the dying person's loved ones about their perceptions of the client's current functioning, recent changes in physical health or behavior, and so forth. Given the possibility of cognitive changes, family miscommunication, and relevant past history, these collateral interviews can take on added importance in end-of-life situations. At some point, it will probably be important to share information with the dying person but it may be useful to conduct at least some of these interviews without the dying person present, so the loved one can be entirely forthright in what she or he says to the counselor.

SYSTEMIC AND ENVIRONMENTAL ISSUES TO BE REVIEWED

The focus of this area is on whether there are any external pressures on the dying person that are affecting her or his mental health, quality of life, and decision making, and, if so, to what extent they can be ameliorated. The "Issues to Consider" document breaks this area into *indirect external coercion* and *direct external coercion*. In terms of *indirect* issues, the document specifies societal conditions and biases that may be leading the person to believe that there are no satisfactory options. This could be because of negative attitudes toward older adults or persons with disabilities. For example, the research indicates that physicians and other people believe that the quality of life of people living with disabilities is significantly worse than the self-ratings by persons living with disabilities themselves (Gill, 2000). The extent to which these negative attitudes influence the ways that health care professionals and significant others treat people who are dying may affect the quality of life of the dying person and her or his own beliefs about herself or himself. Similarly, the lack of societal commitment to maintaining and improving the quality of life of persons who are dying, through adequate funding for and access to health care, trained professional caregivers, appropriate medications, and proper psychosocial support, can lead people to believe that there is little point in trying to stay alive. Therapists who are familiar with care options can provide clients with resources that may help them live higher quality, and perhaps longer, lives.

CASE 10:

William was consulted by Norma when she felt overwhelmed by finding out that her AIDS had progressed and the medication was no longer working. She reported that her physician said he thought she had only a few more months to live but she did not hear much more of what he said because she was in shock. Now, she came in to see William because a friend of hers, who also had HIV disease, said he was knowledgeable about helping people who were dying of AIDS. One of the first things William did was discuss options with Norma and get a release to talk with her physician. When he learned that she did not have any other treatment options, he asked her if she was aware of hospice care. When she said she had heard of it but did not know much about it, William set up a meeting with the hospice team. Afterward, Norma said it sounded good but she did not want to just give up and die. William explained to her that the research indicated that people with certain conditions may actually live longer under hospice care (Connor, Pyenson, Fitch, Spence, & Iwasaki, 2007), perhaps because their symptoms are being treated, which reduces the stress on the body. Norma agreed to give hospice a try, at which point she had to terminate with William and was instead seen by the hospice team for her psychosocial needs. As she was nearing death, she had her nurse call William and he saw her one last time before she died. He attended her funeral a few days later.

The final topic to be explored is *direct external coercion*, which "may be subtle or overt, may be actually occurring or merely a perception of the individual, could occur intentionally or accidentally" (Working Group, 2000, p. 85). The classic examples of coercion are decisions made by health care facilities or insurance companies to limit care in order to save money or other resources. Alternatively, providers may suggest scaling back treatment without providing sufficient explanation, which leads the client to believe that she or he is being abandoned by the health care team. In either case, the counselor may need to take a proactive advocacy role to assist the client in getting the services she or he needs and clearing up any miscommunications.

USE OF ASSESSMENT INSTRUMENTS WITH DYING CLIENTS

Counselors may want to use one or more types of assessment instruments to supplement their own perspective. There are multiple challenges with doing so. First, many instruments have not been validated with physically ill individuals, let alone those who are dying. Thus, the validity of many standard instruments is questionable. Although it is a bit out of date at this point, counselors who are interested in finding some objective assessment instruments that are designed for use with people who are dying can start with the Toolkit of Instruments to Measure End-of-Life Care (www.chcr.brown.edu/pcoc/toolkit.htm). The other issue is the trade-off in cost in time and energy that it will take for the client to complete the instrument versus the benefit for the dying person. Given that time is obviously a precious commodity for the terminally ill individual, the question is whether having the person complete an instrument is the best way to get the information. The counselor will want to be able to make a strong case to the client that the instrument is necessary to helping the client reach her or his goals.

CONCLUSION

Many counselors are not professionally prepared to provide therapy to persons who are near the end of life. Although it can be difficult work, it is also very rewarding, so I hope that counselors will be willing to take the time to learn more about providing this type of counseling. I believe that I have received more from these clients than I have given them. I live my life differently, I appreciate people and time more, and I have worked with some of the more remarkable and resilient people I will ever know.

REFERENCES

Amir, M., & Ramati, A. (2002). Post-traumatic symptoms, emotional distress and quality of life in long-term survivors of breast cancer: A preliminary research. *Journal of Anxiety Disorders, 16*, 195–206.

Ballantyne, J. C. (2007). Opioid misuse in oncology pain patients. *Current Pain and Headache Reports, 11*, 276–282.

Benyamin, R., Trescot, A. M., Datta, S., Buenaventure, R., Adlaka, R., Sehgal, N. et al. (2008). Opioid complications and side effects. *Pain Physician, 11*(Suppl. 2), S105–S120.

Blackhall, L. J., Murphy, S. T., Frank, G., Michel, V., & Azen, S. (1995). Ethnicity and attitudes toward patient autonomy. *Journal of the American Medical Association, 274*, 820–825.

Block, D. D. (2000). Assessing and managing depression in the terminally ill patient. *Annals of Internal Medicine, 132*, 209–218.

Braun, U. K., Kunik, M. E., & Pham, C. (2008). Treating depression in terminally ill patients can optimize their physical comfort at the end of life and provide them the opportunity to confront and prepare for death. *Geriatrics, 63*(6), 25–27.

Breitbart, W., Poppito, S., Rosenfeld, B., Vickers, A. J., Li, Y., Abbey, J. et al. (2012). Pilot randomized controlled trial of individual meaning-centered psychotherapy for patients with advanced cancer. *Journal of Clinical Oncology, 30*, 1304–1309.

Breitbart, W., Rosenfeld, B., Gibson, C., Pessin, H., Poppito, S., Nelson, C. et al. (2010). Meaning-centered group psychotherapy for patients with advanced cancer: A pilot randomized controlled trial. *Psycho-oncology, 19*, 21–28.

Carrese, J. A., & Rhodes, L. A. (1995). Western bioethics on the Navajo reservation. *Journal of the American Medical Association, 274*, 826–829.

Chapple, A., Ziebland, S., McPherson, A., & Herxheimer, A. (2006). What people close to death say about euthanasia and assisted suicide: A qualitative study. *Journal of Medical Ethics, 32*, 706–710.

Chochinov, H. M., Hack, T., Hassard, T., Kristjanson, L. J., McClement, S., & Harlos, M. (2005). Dignity therapy: A novel psychotherapeutic intervention for patients near the end of life. *Journal of Clinical Oncology, 23,* 5520–5525.

Chochinov, H. M., Kristjanson, L. J., Breitbart, W., McClement, S., Hack, T. F., Hassard, T. et al. (2011). Effect of dignity therapy on distress and end-of-life experience in terminally ill patients: A randomized controlled trial. *Lancet Oncology, 12,* 753–762.

Clarke, D. M., Kissane, D. W., Trauer, T., & Smith, G. C. (2005). Demoralization, anhedonia and grief in patients with severe physical illness. *World Psychiatry, 4,* 96–105.

Clayton, J. M., Hancock, K., Parker, S., Butow, P. N., Walder, S., Carrick, S. et al. (2008). Sustaining hope when communicating with terminally ill patients and their families: A systemic review. *Psycho-oncology, 17,* 641–659.

Connor, S. R., Pyenson, B., Fitrch, K., Spence, C., & Iwasaki, K. (2007). Comparing hospice and nonhospice patient survival among patients who die within a three-year window. *Journal of Pain and Symptom Management, 33,* 238–246.

Dharia, S., Verilla, K., & Breden, E. L. (2011). The 3 D's of geriatric psychiatry: Depression, delirium, and dementia. *The Consultant Pharmacist, 26,* 566–578.

Emanuel, E. J., Fairclough, D. L., Slutsman, J., & Emanuel, L. L. (2000). Understanding economic and other burdens of terminal illness: The experience of patients and their caregivers. *Annals of Internal Medicine, 132,* 451–459.

Enyert, G., & Burman, M. E. (1999). A qualitative study of self-transcendence in caregivers of terminally ill patients. *American Journal of Hospice and Palliative Care, 16,* 455–463.

Flood, M., & Buckwalter, K. C. (2009a). Recommendations for mental health care of older adults: Part 2—An overview of dementia, delirium, and substance abuse. *Journal of Gerontological Nursing, 35,* 35–47.

Flood, M., & Buckwalter, K. C. (2009b). Recommendations for mental health care of older adults: Part 2—An overview of depression and anxiety. *Journal of Gerontological Nursing, 35,* 26–34.

Ganzini, L., Goy, E. R., & Dobscha, S. K. (2008). Why Oregon patients request assisted death: Family members' views. *Journal of General Internal Medicine, 23,* 154–157.

Ganzini, L., Goy, E. R., & Dobscha, S. K. (2009). Oregonian's reasons for requesting physician aid in dying. *Archives of Internal Medicine, 169,* 489–492.

Gill, C. J. (2000). Health professionals, disability, and assisted suicide: An examination of relevant empirical evidence and reply to Batavia. *Psychology, Public Policy, and Law, 6,* 526–545.

Graziottin, A., Gardner-Nix, J., Stumpf, M., & Berliner, M. N. (2011). Opioids: How to improve compliance and adherence. *Pain Practice, 11,* 574–581.

Grisso, T., & Appelbaum, P. S. (1998). *Assessing competence to consent to treatment: A guide for physicians and other health care professionals.* New York: Oxford.

Gutheil, T. G. (1985). Medicolegal pitfalls in the treatment of borderline patients. *American Journal of Psychiatry, 142,* 9–14.

Himmelstein, D. U., Thorne, D., Warren, E., & Woolhandler, S. (2009). Medical bankruptcy in the United States, 2007: Results of a national study. *American Journal of Medicine, 122,* 741–746.

Johnson, S. (2007). Hope in terminal illness: An evolutionary concept analysis. *International Journal of Palliative Nursing, 13,* 451–459.

Kolva, E., Rosenfeld, B., Pessin, H., Breitbart, W., & Brescia, R. (2011). Anxiety in terminally ill cancer patients. *Journal of Pain and Symptom Management, 42,* 691–701.

Lippe, P. M., Brock, C., David, J., Crossno, R., & Gitlow, S. (2010). The First National pain Medicine Summit—Final summary report. *Pain Medicine, 11,* 1447–1468.

Malhi, G. S., Adams, D., Porter, R., Wignall, A., Lampe, L., O'Connor, N. et al. (2009). Clinical practice recommendations for depression. *Acta Psychiatrica Scandinavica, 11*(Suppl., 439), 8–26.

McClain, C. S., Rosenfeld, B., & Breitbartm, W. (2003). Effect of spiritual well-being on end-of-life despair in terminally-ill cancer patients. *Lancet, 361,* 1603–1607.

Muskin, P. R. (1998). The request to die: Role for a psychodynamic perspective on physician-assisted suicide. *Journal of the Australian Mathematical Society, 279,* 323–328.

Noorani, N. H., & Montagnini, M. (2007). Recognizing depression in palliative care patients. *Journal of Palliative Medicine, 10,* 458–464.

Orr, K., & Taylor, D. (2007). Psychostimulants in the treatment of depression: A review of the evidence. *CNS Drugs, 21,* 239–257.

Rosenfeld, B., Breitbart, W., Gibson, C., Kramer, M., Tomarken, A., Nelson, C. et al. (2006). Desire for hastened death among patients with advanced AIDS. *Psychosomatics, 47,* 504–512.

Rosenfeld, B., Gibson, C., Kramer, M., & Breitbart, W. (2004). Hopelessness and terminal illness: The construct of hopelessness in patients with advanced AIDS. *Palliative & Supportive Care, 2,* 43–53.

Rosenfeld, B., Pessin, H., Lewis, C., Abbey, J., Olden, M., Sachs, E. et al. (2011). Assessing hopelessness in terminally ill cancer patients: Development of the Hopelessness Assessment in Illness Questionnaire. *Psychological Assessment, 23,* 325–336.

Stravynski, A., & Boyer, R. (2001). Loneliness in relation to suicide ideation and parasuicide: A population-wide study. *Suicide and Life-Threatening Behavior, 31,* 32–40.

Theeke, L. A., Goins, R. T., Moore, J., & Campbell, H. (2012). Loneliness, depression, social support, and quality of life in older chronically ill Appalachians. *Journal of Psychology, 146,* 155–171.

Trimpey, M., & Davidson, S. (1998). Nursing care of personality disorders in the medical surgery setting. *Nursing Clinics of North America, 33,* 173–186.

Wein, S., Sulkes, A., & Stemmer, S. (2010). The oncologist's role in managing depression, anxiety, and demoralization with advanced cancer. *Cancer Journal, 16,* 493–499.

Werth, J. L., Jr. (1999). Mental health professionals and assisted death: Perceived ethical obligations and proposed guidelines for practice. *Ethics & Behavior, 9,* 159–183.

Werth, J. L., Jr., Gordon, J. R., & Johnson, R. R., Jr. (2002). Psychosocial issues near the end of life. *Aging & Mental Health, 6,* 402–412.

Working Group on Assisted Suicide and End-of-Life Decisions. (2000). *Report to the Board of Directors of the American Psychological Association.* Washington, DC: American Psychological Association. Available at http://www.apa.org/pubs/info/reports/aseol-full.pdf

6

Lifespan Considerations for People Who Are Near the End of Life

ILLENE NOPPE CUPIT, DEIRDRE M. RADOSEVICH,
AND GAIL E. TRIMBERGER

One of the authors of this chapter encountered the following as a hospice social worker:

> **CASE 1:**
>
> Edward was an 80-year-old Native American man who had never been married. He had end-stage cardiac disease and was being cared for in the home of his 24-year-old nephew. When Edward's brothers would visit, they followed their tribe's traditional customs for a dying person. This included covering Edward with a ceremonial robe and laying an eagle feather near his head. When the brothers would leave, the nephew removed the items with little regard for their traditional meaning. It was important for the professional counseling staff to assess this cultural difference and adapt their behaviors accordingly.

What can be discerned from this brief scenario? Clearly the counseling staff were required to juggle the needs of a dying elderly patient with those of a young adult caregiving family member. In addition, there was another "ball up in the air" involving two cultural contexts: traditional Native American rituals competing with a young adult's contemporary approach to ministering to the dying. Understanding dying from a lifespan perspective, therefore, encompasses learning about a complex process involving developmental, social, and cultural factors.

End-of-life concerns usually are associated with middle and old age, but the sad reality is that younger people may also find themselves coping with their mortality because of a life-threatening illness, genetic defect, or a traumatic injury. The process of dying has no age constraints. Merely using chronological age as the anchor for understanding how dying is perceived and treated misses the rich confluence of factors that make up the ecological lifespace of all of the involved participants in this end-of-life journey.

The developmental perspective, which considers age-related tasks within a social–ecological context, allows one to better conceptualize the multifaceted issues people face when coping with end-of-life issues—whether that be everyday issues occurring in the home or school context to coping with painful medical procedures, multiple medical providers, and even separation from loved ones, or requirements to make end-of-life decisions. It is important to remember that the dying person is still a person who may be expected to continue with daily responsibilities such as completing homework or caring for others.

Each period of development has its unique tasks and concerns, but there also are several issues that cut across the life span. These are:

1. *The cultural and personal meanings that are attached to the dying process.* Every social group has a "death system" (Kastenbaum, 1972) that provides structural and culturally agreed upon constructions of what dying, death, and mortality mean to its members. In addition to symbols and objects related to the end of life, the death system prescribes how the dying are to be cared for and treated—the support system. Such prescriptions also involve the social roles of the dying in terms of their rights and expectations. Contemporary Western cultures frequently are referred to as "death phobic," which may lead to the social isolation of the dying by friends and family. Because social support has been found to be crucial for managing life-threatening conditions, such "social death" may compound the complications of the dying process at each phase of the life span.
2. *The tasks of dying.* Since the publication of the groundbreaking work of Kübler-Ross (1969) presenting dying as a graduated movement through five stages, the end of life has been viewed as occurring in phases, dual processes, and stages of varying numbers. The task approach, promoted by Corr (1992), posits that the dying have certain needs (i.e., biological, spiritual, social, and psychological), which should be met in order for the dying process to be managed. The types of tasks, and the degree of their relative importance, may change at different points in the life span because they intersect with the normative developmental tasks of each phase. Also shaping this developmental-dying task approach is the course of the illness itself, or its "dying trajectory" (Glaser & Strauss, 1965). In this case, we wish to know how people and their loved ones manage when there is lingering dying with much uncertainty, remissions and reappearances of the life-threatening illnesses, and slow or rapid declines in status. The issue is how self- and other attributions change depending upon the age of the person who is dying as the dying process proceeds in its predictable or unpredictable course.

3. *Dying as a response to the confluence of developmental, social, and institutional/cultural factors.* Figure 6.1 represents a summation of how the death system and tasks of dying and developmental phases overlap to create the unique environment and phenomenology of the person who is coping with his or her dying. It highlights that the dying experience can take on a myriad of forms and meanings for the dying person and his or her loved ones. Effective counseling must bear in mind how these factors represent the sum total of the dying experience and underscore the fact that dying is not a solitary affair at any age. Looking broadly at the normative lifespan tasks will therefore help to illuminate the end-of-life issues within the context of human development.

CHILDREN AND ADOLESCENTS AND THE END OF LIFE

The Death System

In the United States and other industrialized countries, the prevailing belief of the death system is that babies and children grow up to outlive their parents. In 2010, the infant mortality rate, or deaths per 1,000 live births in these nations (e.g., the United States, New Zealand, Norway, Japan), averaged to about 5, whereas in the least developed countries (e.g., Afghanistan, Angola, Central African Republic, Somalia), the average is 44 (U.N. Interagency Group on Child Mortality Estimation, 2011). Thus, there is a different

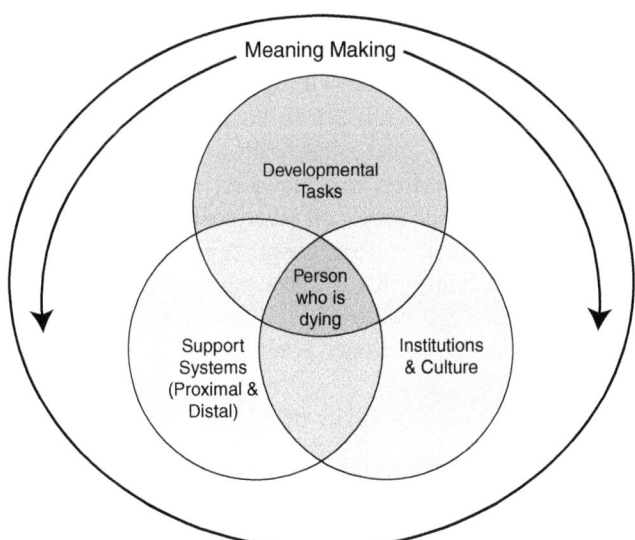

FIGURE 6.1
Dying as the Confluence of Development, Support Systems, and Institutions

set of expectations and beliefs about dying children, although the support system may not find it any less painful. In these least developed countries, childhood dying occurs because of the ravages of infectious disease, food shortages, and trauma associated with war. For adolescents, the prevalence of dying from HIV/AIDS, work-related accidents, and homicide increase substantially, particularly for men (Noppe & Noppe, 2009).

In the United States, however, according to the National Center for Health Statistics (Murphy, Xu, & Kochanek, 2012), the leading cause of death for U.S. children aged 1 to 14 is accidents (primarily motor vehicle accidents). For adolescents older than age 14, motor vehicle accidents and homicides were the predominant causes of death. Although it is true that such accidents frequently lead to a quick dying trajectory, the outcomes may also lead to the equally heartbreaking situation of a youngster placed on life support for an indefinite period of time (Noppe & Noppe, 2009). As is true for their elders, advances in medicine enable medical personnel to sustain life (but not, perhaps, its quality) for infants, children, and adolescents. In these cases, loved ones may have to choose either to continue sustaining life in the face of medical futility in spite of potential irreversible developmental delays of some sort, or ending the life of a young person—an act that is anathema to Western ways of thinking and its death system. Research suggests that physicians typically are reluctant to stop aggressive treatment and would be more amenable to referring children to pediatric hospice care sooner if they were allowed to continue curative treatment (Fowler et al., 2006).

Physicians and parents alike view recommendations for pediatric hospice as "giving up hope" (Dickens, 2010; Fowler et al., 2006), which can lead to a poorer quality death experience for the child and the family. According to a study involving the withdrawal of life support for pediatric patients (Zawistowski & DeVita, 2004), such decisions were made after extensive stays in intensive care units, with a median hospital stay of 20 days and most of the children quickly died once the life support was removed. The patients in this study all were suffering from life-threatening illnesses with the process of ending life-sustaining intervention involving medical personnel and family. It is frustrating that no studies to date have looked at similar issues for children who suffer from a traumatic injury because of accidents as its prevalence is relatively high for adolescents.

The Tasks of Dying

Most of what is known about the living–dying interval for children comes from a relatively extensive literature on pediatric oncology patients (Walsh, 2010). Walsh poignantly describes how coping with the devastating consequences of childhood cancer involves an emotional roller coaster for patients and their families. The decision-making process of moving from curative to palliative treatments involves psychological fortitude that is hard to imagine.

The tasks of dying involve the fulfillment of more than the alleviation of pain and meeting basic biological functions. For the dying child, fear of separation may be more primary than fear of dying. Multiple hospital stays and seclusion from family can be particularly difficult for an infant or young child because of his or her limited verbal abilities. Older children and adolescents are also separated from their peers, who play such a central role in mastering normative developmental tasks.

Adolescents with life-threatening illnesses also must cope with changes in body image, loss of independence, little privacy, changed relationships with parents and siblings, and lack of intimacy, which they crave from boyfriends or girlfriends (Stevens, Dunsmore, Bennett, & Young, 2009).

CASE 2:

Alan was approaching his 21st birthday when he was referred to palliative care for a life-limiting genetic condition. Although his biological age was 20, he presented much younger as is often the case for youth who have lived with a chronic illness much of their lives. Much to the dismay of his parents, Alan's biggest concern was living until his birthday so he could "legally drink." As his condition worsened, he had no appetite for alcohol, but he did not waiver from this as his primary goal. The second challenge for Alan's parents came when he needed physical assistance for his bathing and toileting needs and expressly did not want his mother to aid him. For most of his life, Alan's mother was his primary caregiver. Although she understood his discomfort having a woman help with such personal care, she felt rejected as his mother and struggled to figure out her new role.

There also is the isolation of communication, described by the groundbreaking work of Bluebond-Langner (1978) who found that terminally ill children frequently used the surrounding physical and social context to indirectly learn about their incurable prognoses. It is hard to tend to the psychological, spiritual, and social needs of pediatric patients in a closed communicative context. Adolescents, who obviously are capable of understanding their illness and extent of trauma (unless they are in a persistent vegetative state), can have their autonomy and identity needs met by being involved in treatment decisions (Freyer, 2004).

CASE 3:

Involving children in their own life and death decisions can be difficult for adults. However, doing so can have a life-changing impact on the surviving parents. One of the authors facilitated a support group for grieving parents. As part of the grieving process, the parents would repeatedly re-live the events of their child's death. In virtually all situations, the parents who allowed their children to participate in treatment decisions found some comfort in their grief knowing they made choices based on their child's desires. One couple, whose 10-year-old daughter had a congenital heart condition, was faced with the decision of having her undergo another heart transplant. They were in conflict about making the conscious choice to put her through the intense pain and recovery process when the outcome was uncertain. Their daughter boldly approached the subject with them and asked for no more surgeries. After ensuring that the girl understood the ramifications of declining surgery, they conceded to her wishes. After her death, when the parents would question the decision they made, they found solace in knowing they granted their daughter's wish versus decided based on their own needs.

Dying as a Confluence

Thus, counseling children, adolescents, and their loved ones depends upon how open the culture and community is to acknowledging a "premature" end of life and whether there are support systems in place (e.g., governmental, community-based, faith-based) to help families and their children. When death systems are overwhelmed, as in rampant death because of war and HIV/AIDS in sub-Saharan Africa or in the inner cities of the United States, the breakdown of the "confluence" leads to significant mental health problems for a traumatized population (Demmer, 2009). Intervention needs to take into consideration the entire ecological system in order to be helpful (Gupta, 2008).

EMERGING ADULTS, YOUNG ADULTS, AND THE END OF LIFE

The Death System

During the 20th century, descriptions of development during adulthood alluded to early, middle, and older phases, following the sequence described by Erik Erikson's (1968) theory of psychosocial development. Such divisions are social constructions and thus are embedded with cultural meanings. Although youth is celebrated in Western societies, there still are cultures (as found in many Native American tribes and in the East) that value their older adults who can remain fully integrated in their families and community roles. However, cultural homogenization has grown out of the importing of Western values through the mass media. The rapid pace of global technological advances has led to a general devaluation of those in the middle-age years and beyond. Furthermore, Arnett (2000) has proposed the existence of a new period of adulthood, "emerging adulthood," for individuals between 18 and 24 years of age.

Emerging adults are characterized by their transitional lifestyles in terms of residence and education, lack of role constraints, experimentation with the job world, and their penchant for identity exploration and self-focus. Despite the potential of death occurrences because of accidents, suicides, homicides, military action, and life-threatening diseases, dying and death are not part of the vocabulary associated with emerging and young adults. Thus, dying is not discussed or acknowledged, and the death system still lacks the "machinery" to accommodate such occurrences. However, with a large young veteran population, many have had to deal with watching their peers and friends die and they might be facing life-threatening maladies themselves. Specifically, coping with the stress of multiple deployments, higher incidents of substance use, and complications from injuries put these veterans at risk for higher incidents of long-term stress-related illnesses and death.

It is always a shock and newsworthy when death does happen to a young adult. We only have to recall the highly publicized case of Terri Schiavo (Gostin, 2005), a woman who at age 26 experienced cardiac arrest and descended into a persistent vegetative state, to bring awareness to our understanding that people face dying in their 20s. In addition, young adults may become involved in caring for their dying grandparents and parents, or know of someone who is facing life-threatening situations from illness or traumatic injury. Research on college student grief has consistently shown that almost half of a college student body has suffered the loss of a loved one within a 24-month period prior to being surveyed. A number of those losses were preceded by a period of physical debilitation of the deceased prior to death (Cupit, Servaty-Seib, Parikh, Walker, & Martin, in process).

Life expectancies vary across the globe, but it is generally true that in most societies the young adult population is its healthiest. However, war, disease, and accidents have had devastating effects on young adult populations in many parts of the world. For example, in South Africa, whole segments of the emerging and young adult population are absent because of the high death rate as a result of AIDS. Their children are raising their siblings, or the grieving (and frequently ill) parents—the children's grandparents—of the deceased are stepping in as parents. Sobering statistics indicate that nearly one in three women aged 25 to 29, and one in four men aged 30 to 34 are HIV positive (Avert, International HIV and AIDS Charity, 2011). In the Middle East, war has ravaged the adult population, with over 600,000 Iraqi deaths after the invasion of March 2003. Most of these deaths, resulting from violent means, are of men aged 15 to 44 years (Burnham, Doocy, Dzeng, Lafta, & Roberts, 2006).

When there is massive and unchecked death that taxes psychological, social, and economic resources, as seen in the examples above, the death system, which evolves over time and relies on cultural institutions and meanings to function effectively, can break down. A consequence of this death system dysfunction may be significant challenges to the traditional coping strategies and support systems of emerging and young adults.

The Tasks of Dying

Learning how to make one's own decisions, constructing and building future life plans, and developing relationships are the major concerns of emerging and young adults. The process of dying can have a significant impact on these normative developmental tasks. It is rare for a young adult, unless involved in military action, to have designated a power of attorney for health care or other type of advance directive. Statistics on completed advance directives by age are hard to come by, but the most recent statistics found for those who were in a nursing home, hospice, or home health care who filed legal end-of-life documents report that they were likely to be 65 years of age or older (Jones, Moss, & Harris-Kojetin, 2011). However, the landmark court cases regarding the withdrawal of life support (e.g., Karen Ann Quinlan, Nancy Cruzan, and recently Terri Schiavo) involved young adults—*not* older adults (Capron, 2007). Even if emerging and young adults do fill out an advance directive, their wishes may be or may not be heeded if medical personnel, finding it difficult to "let go" of a young patient, argue that continued aggressive treatment is the best course of action.

Social needs are at the forefront, but dying young adults might find that their good friends and significant others may abandon them out of their own discomfort and dismay over the thought of dying (Cook & Oltjenbruns, 1998). Physical comfort or treatments may also be sacrificed if it means increased hair loss, bloating, or other insults to a positive body image. The workplace and school are notorious for poor or nonexistent policies regarding leaves of absence or flexible schedules during the management of the disease process. All of this occurs at a time when career building and degree seeking should be taking place, leading to additional psychological and social distress.

CASE 4:

Twenty-two-year-old Sandra, newly married, lived in Florida when she was diagnosed with cancer. Sandra's parents begged her to come home so they could care for her. Her husband of less than 1 year stayed in Florida to work while Sandra returned to her parents' home in the Midwest until her death. Sandra's cancer was very invasive requiring surgeries that disfigured her neck and shoulder, accompanied by severe edema of one arm. Part of her decision to remain in her parents' home was based on these physical changes in her appearance. She felt unattractive and did not want her husband to see her in that state. Although Sandra had her physical needs met and was in the home of her choice, she was emotionally torn by the decision to be apart from her new husband. Because of the distance, Sandra's husband was not present when she died and was unable to receive adequate support from the counseling staff.

Dying as a Confluence

If we view the experience of dying as the intersection of institutions, support systems, and the person's attributes (physical, psychological, and social), we can see how difficult it is to make sense of dying (the meaning making) during these years. From a Western perspective, the years of emerging adulthood and young adulthood represent peak physical beauty, strength, energy, sexuality, intellectual capacity, and a future orientation—"You have your whole life ahead of you!" This cultural mantra must be reconciled with the debilitating effects of disease, loss of the future and its associated plan making, and a pervasive sense of helplessness.

Institutional mechanisms reward aggressive treatments and a medical bureaucracy that is difficult for young adults to negotiate on their own. Young adults, whose major developmental task involves independence from their family of origin, might have no recourse but to turn to their parents for help. Social support may be difficult to come by as threatened friends and family back away from their ill loved one, especially if there is misdirected anger.

CASE 5:

John and his wife moved in with John's parents so they could aid in the caregiving when John was in the final stages of cancer. This situation was successful in providing support for both John and his new, young wife. Yet, there were frequent times when John's wife and his mother had role conflicts, putting John in the role of mediator between the two women. The counselor's role is to help the family find ways to resolve their conflicts without burdening the dying patient whose energy is limited.

When death enters the home, emerging and young adults face many challenges. Their needs may not be met by the intersection of personal, relational, and institutional systems. For example, across the globe, young adults who are dying from a stigmatized disease such as AIDS, or wounds from civil strife, are left abandoned with little medicine or support. Another example might be seen in young married couples who may find sexual intimacy difficult to enjoy and who have no one to turn to for help in this matter. In households with young children, ailing parents who are physically and emotionally uncomfortable, might find that they have a short fuse when it comes to living with the usual tantrums and defiance typical of their children. Such problems may be exacerbated by economic stressors and isolation from extended family.

Further, we should not neglect those young adults who are caring for loved ones who are dying. Romm (2009) in her memoir, openly described her own journey as she comes home from school to help (and watch) her once-vibrant mother die from cancer. Although she bravely works at being supportive of her mother and father through the disease process, her own developmental needs get in the way, understandably leading her down an angry and depressed path.

Contrary to the "stage" described by Kübler-Ross (1969), denial may be an effective coping strategy to maintain relationships and to achieve some semblance of quality of life (Feifel, 1977). The downside, however, is that such denial may prohibit using palliative and hospice care when it can be helpful at this time. The National Hospice and Palliative Care Organization (2010) reported that, as of 2009, children, adolescents, and young adults made up less than 1% of the hospice care population.

Thus, there is much room for improvement for young adults who are dying or for those who are involved with loved ones who are dying. One unexpected place where support might be possible is through the use of social media, which can offer information, support groups, and an opportunity to blog about one's experiences (Sofka, Cupit, & Gilbert, 2012).

MIDDLE AGE AND DYING

The Death System

In contemporary Western societies, increasing life expectancies has led to attributions given to the men and women in their 40s, 50s, and 60s. Erikson (1968) characterized this as a period of "generativity vs. stagnation." By this he meant that the main developmental tasks involved achievement, making creations of lasting value, and mentoring the younger generation. Of course, the prior developmental tasks of identity and intimacy are also present, but there is a sense of urgency that all of those wonderful plans and projects must bear fruit now and can no longer be deferred. Neugarten and Datan (1973), drawing upon the Eriksonian notion of identity crisis, posited that during midlife there was a reorientation in an individual's perspective from "time since birth" to "time left to live." Thus, the death system acknowledges that the "mid-life crisis" involves meanings and systems in place to support the idea that midlifers must work hard to avoid death before all of those plans are realized.

CASE 6:

Lori, in her late 40s, married with one college-aged daughter, was referred to hospice with advanced cancer. During the first meeting with the hospice staff, Lori exhibited restlessness and very high levels of anxiety. These symptoms were initially viewed as responses to pain (which Lori also experienced). However, as the symptoms became increasingly difficult to medically manage, the role of the professional staff was to explore the root of her anxiety. Through intense listening and observation, it became apparent that Lori was most proud of her career accomplishments. Her role in the work place provided her with her strongest sense of identity. Up to this point, the family had been hovering and protecting her from external stimuli. Lori's anxiety lessened when her family recognized (and supported) Lori's need to go to the office, if only for short periods of time.

Because the leading causes of death during this period are the result of heart disease and cancer, such deaths are viewed as "losing the battle" after a "courageous war" has been fought. In order to prevent such "wars" to begin with, midlifers are expected to be "youthful." "Acting your age" no longer has meaning when life expectancies keep on increasing and there is a strong cultural push for active and engaged lifestyles. Given that the number of deaths increase during midlife, the components and functions of the death system (e.g., health care personnel, facial creams promising a youthful glow, will preparation) are fairly well established. However, it is important to recognize that death systems vary by culture, and thus those who might be perceived as a youthful middle-aged person in one society may be viewed as an elder in another.

By interviewing Black and Afrikaans women in South Africa, for example, one of the authors learned that two women of the same age had different perspectives on their developmental status, with the Black woman, who worked on the janitorial staff of a major university, calling herself old whereas the Afrikaans secretary described herself as young and vigorous. Both of these South African women were concerned about caring for their elderly mothers, which also is an experience common to those in middle age. Accordingly, many middle agers see their parents through their dying process and experience an increasing number of dying friends and relatives. Contemplating death in the future no longer is an abstraction for people at midlife.

The Tasks of Dying and Dying as a Confluence

It is difficult to separate the tasks of dying from the confluence model when describing dying during the midlife years. Perhaps this is because, in a number of respects, the intersection of institutional, social, and individual systems with meeting physical needs (e.g., controlling pain), psychological needs (e.g., maintaining autonomy and a quality life), social needs (e.g., preserving social relationships), and spiritual needs (e.g., making sense of one's life within a larger, more cosmic context) seems most functional for people at midlife. In Western societies, although being stricken with a life-threatening disease for those who are in their 40s through 60s may be considered premature, it does not have the connotations of tragedy and injustice that is associated with dying at younger ages. For those who are at a relatively comfortable junction in life, institutional supports, as found in health care, estate and legal planning, as well as religious institutions, respond well to midlifers, who are seen as competent and capable of making autonomous decisions. Hopefully, they have health care insurance, resources to get information such as through the Internet, and the motivation to actively participate in their treatment. For example, it is more common for middle-age people to use hospice care, and so the hospice teams might be more experienced and knowledgeable about how to support and care for people at this stage of life.

Many midlifers also are well-connected in their interpersonal relationships. They may be in a long-term marriage or relationship and thus have someone who can help with their needed care, their children are most likely to be adults who can help out, and friends and coworkers may be available to pitch in with meal preparation or shoveling a driveway. Of course, individual factors will play an important role in this confluence of the dying process. A positive, optimistic attitude also seems to be an important element in extending quality of life (Roberts, Kuncel, Shiner, Caspi, & Goldberg, 2007). Dying persons who have mental health problems or financial worries, are socially isolated, or lack the resources to negotiate our complex health and legal systems lack the support that is necessary for "dying well."

OLDER ADULTS AND THE END OF LIFE

The Death System

In societies where life expectancies have extended well into old age, the largest proportion of deaths occur for older adults. For example, the most recent published U.S. mortality statistics (2007) clearly show that with age, the number deaths increase. For example, the U.S. Centers for Disease Control and Prevention reported that there were 389,238 deaths for the 65- to 74-year-old cohort, increasing to 713,647 deaths for the 85 years and over cohort (Murphy et al., 2012). Coupled with our glorification of youth, this close association between death and advanced age fosters a devaluing of older adults in many Westernized countries—an attitude that many fear leads to less than optimal care for a dying older adult.

This attitude may even be assumed by older adults themselves, and their level of expectation of quality treatment from others during their dying may be low. Whereas young and middle-age adults may be exhorted to play the social role of sick person as a tragic hero—a brave fighter and warrior–the social role of sick person for older adults may be of passive, almost child-like acceptance and resignation. If an old person plays this role well, caregivers may mistake his or her depression as being "ready to die" (Kastenbaum, 2012). Many components of the death system (i.e., people, places, symbols) are involved in the important function of ministering to the dying, but a culturally supported aversion to those who are old can result in their social isolation and neglect at a time when dying older adults also are more likely to be frail and dependent upon others for their basic care (Lunney, Lynn, Foley, Lipson, & Guralnik, 2003).

The Tasks of Dying

Regardless of health status, meeting the biological, psychological, social, and spiritual needs of older adults can take significant energy. Maintaining a sense of integrity in facing death in one's last years of life becomes challenging when there is functional decline with a course of dying that is lingering. In addition to pain management, meeting physical needs may involve basic routine care, including diapering. Self-esteem can decrease when physical grooming is neglected. Even the simple act of taking an elderly woman for a haircut and styling, with perhaps some application of makeup, can lift spirits in untold ways. The American Cancer Society recognizes this need with their "Look Good ... Feel Better" program. (Fishlinger, 2010). Although we mention such support for physical appearance in this section on older adults, such programs are really targeted for all ages.

Whereas it is easy to acknowledge that younger women desire to look physically attractive despite their life-threatening illness, we should not neglect these needs for older women. Dying does not necessarily preclude wanting to look good for any age, but this want might be especially unnoticed for older adults. When one of the authors had such an outing with her mother-in-law who was living with Alzheimer's, the older woman became less confused for the remainder of the day. It should be noted that taking some individuals with Alzheimer's out of their environment, regardless of the purpose of the outing, can increase confusion. Therefore, if an outing is not advisable because of the individual's level of cognitive functioning, there are other creative ways to bring these services to the home.

The same is true for the social, psychological, and spiritual needs, which truly are tested in the face of "social death." Losing friends and siblings, moving away from home, and seeing family who live afar only periodically, disrupt long-term social ties that impart a sense of history when a person is confronting dying and death. An activity that might help is to encourage older people who are dying to participate in a "life review" (Chochinov, 2006). When the process works, it enables an individual to engage in *meaning-making*, or an integrative coherence to one's life story as well as its ultimate end. When this process is facilitated with compassionate care, it can do much to alleviate some of the anxiety and depression associated with increased disability, dependence, and a sense of isolation (Chochinov, 2006).

CASE 7:

Robert was in his mid-70s when he was diagnosed with cancer. He had three sons from a previous marriage and lived with his second wife who was experiencing some signs of dementia. As a young man, Robert had served in the military. He had been retired for some years from a very successful and prominent executive position. Even in the final stages of his cancer, Robert was resistant to help from others, holding on to his strong sense of independence. During visits with the counselor, Robert would align the chairs as if he were being interviewed by a reporter. Conversations were filled with stories of his accomplishments and successes. Recognizing Robert's need to maintain control of his situation much as he did in his executive role, the counselor suggested he may wish to write his own obituary. This proved to be a very effective intervention, fulfilling his need for life review and ensuring that he was able to tell his own story. Once the obituary was written and given to his family with specific instructions, Robert was able to relax and allow others to care for him and his wife.

This life review not only meets psychological needs, it can help to alleviate the spiritual and existential crises that face many older dying patients who may reach back to earlier religious teachings or have a reawakened "soul-searching" to help explain their suffering and anticipation of the afterlife. Such was found by McClain, Rosenfeld, and Breitbart (2003) who studied cancer patients toward the end of their lives. Those participants who maintained a sense of "spiritual well-being" seemed to fare better in terms of an attenuated sense of end-of-life despair.

Such holistic care for the dying is necessary at any point of the life span, but societal devaluation and the normative difficulties of old age may make this goal particularly difficult to meet. In more impoverished nations with scarce resources, it is enough of a test to meet basic physical needs and find necessary medication. In African nations decimated by AIDS, there may not be family members left to take care of the dying older loved ones. Similarly, few may be available to provide palliative services for the old and infirm. As Chochinov (2006) eloquently states, "... patients must not only be made to feel more comfortable, but more broadly, provided with comfort" (p. 84).

TABLE 6.1
Summary of Lifespan Considerations for People Near the End of Life

Developmental Period	Selected Normative Developmental Tasks/Achievements	Challenges of Dying	Strategies to Facilitate Coping
Infancy	Attachment, Language Development, Attain fine and gross motor skills, develop sense of self, emotional and body regulation.	Fear of separation from loved ones; becoming avoidant of touch, disruption of routines, contending with unfamiliar environments, loss of developmental milestones.	-Focus is on the needs of adults rather than the infant's attachment needs. -Finding resources for respite care for caregivers. -Encourage the guardians to pre-plan for funeral and other end-of-life decisions. -Encourage creation of memorial items: footprint, lock of hair, etc. -Provide education on dying process, in accordance with client's level of readiness. -Assess and explore spiritual and cultural beliefs and needs.
Childhood	Peer development; become more independent from family; language, concept, and motor development; self-esteem development; creation of a positive body image; learning how to function in groups and educational environments.	Conceptual understanding of dying, fear of separation, isolation from peers, coping with medical treatments, being treated as a "normal" child at home and at school, maintaining a sense of independence.	-Involve in treatment decisions, appropriate to child's level of understanding and in accordance with the child's level of readiness. -If given permission, educate school personnel and other social supports. -Encourage expression of feelings through creative means: play, art, etc. -Establish safe places where the child does not have to receive invasive procedures, be "different", etc. -Provide education on dying process to level of understanding and readiness. - Assess and explore spiritual and cultural beliefs and needs.

(Continued)

TABLE 6.1
Summary of Lifespan Considerations for People Near the End of Life (*Continued*)

Developmental Period	Selected Normative Developmental Tasks/Achievements	Challenges of Dying	Strategies to Facilitate Coping
Adolescence	Independence from family, developing a sense of identity, learning how to interact with the other sex, developing a positive sense of self and body, coping with the changes associated with puberty, exploring sexuality, developing future goals and plans.	Understanding the disease and treatments, loss of peers, coping with disruptions in physical development, dealing with absences and re-entries into school, feeling physically unattractive (e.g., hair loss), planning for a curtailed future. Loss of functions if in a traumatic injury.	-Encourage continued involvement in "adolescent" activities, as tolerated. -With permission, offer education to peers, school personnel, and other social supports to minimize withdrawal based on fears. -Involve adolescent in treatment and care decisions. -Encourage expression of feelings through creative means: art, prose, music, etc. -Provide education on dying process. -Assess and explore spiritual and cultural beliefs and needs.
Emerging & Young Adulthood	Crystallization of an identity, developing intimate relationships, setting up own household, educational pursuits leading to career development, contending with transitions in personal, educational and occupational pursuits, starting a family.	Maintaining intimacy and sexuality, finding one's place in the adult world with a threatened future, continuing in career development, coping with educational and job disruption, contending with increased dependency, coping with urging "not to give up," concerns with family planning. Loss of functions if traumatically injured.	-Encourage conversations regarding advance directives. -Facilitate group meetings for family and other social supports to minimize potential conflicts and maximize understanding. -Provide education on dying process. -Provide support and education for sexual intimacy, if faced with physical limitations. -Assess and explore spiritual and cultural beliefs and needs.

Middle Age	Developing a sense of generativity in work and interpersonal relationships, taking care of adolescent children and elderly parents, integrating a shifting perspective on the developmental time line and associated reevaluation of the self, planning for retirement.	Coping with the dying of peers and parents, developing legacies or aspects of the self of lasting value, making treatment decisions for self or others, concerns with financial planning, loss of independence.	-Encourage pre-planning for funeral and other end-of-life decisions. -Offer resources for other commitments (e.g., caring for elderly parents, etc.). -Encourage life review. -Encourage creation of legacy for children, grandchildren, etc. -Encourage conversations regarding advance directives. -Provide education on dying process. - Provide support and education for sexual intimacy, if faced with physical limitations. - Assess and explore spiritual and cultural beliefs and needs.
Older Adulthood	Developing a sense of integrity for entire life course, engaging in life review for meaning making, remaining active and engaged in society and in social networks, following a healthy life style in order to maintain quality of life, maintaining or creating a philosophy of one's own life cycle.	Maintaining quality of life in face of debilitation, preserving a sense of dignity, coping with social isolation, contending with moving into an institution, preserving a positive sense of self in the face of physical decline, participating in end-of-life decision making, finding social support to provide physical and medical assistance in addition to daily living assistance (especially important when there is dementia).	-Encourage life review. -Include in all conversations regardless of perceived cognitive abilities. -Allow to make own decisions to extent possible. -Encourage pre-planning for funeral and other end-of-life decisions. -Support desire for independence while offering resources for ADL assistance. -Encourage conversations regarding advance directives. -Provide education on dying process. - Provide support and education for sexual intimacy, if faced with physical limitations. - Assess and explore spiritual and cultural beliefs and needs.

The Confluence Model

Many have tried to define what is meant by a "good death." Westernized approaches herald dying in one's sleep, in one's bed at home, at a ripe old age. Kastenbaum (2004) elaborated by specifying that in addition to the needs associated with tasks of dying, a good death affirms our sense of personal value, relationships, coherence, and reflects the anticipated end of a good life. Chochinov (2006) underscored that a good death involves maintaining a sense of dignity. Dignity is fostered when a dying person's self-worth is upheld by social and societal support. It requires the confluence of personal, institutional, and social factors and is particularly important for societies facing increased numbers of aging citizens. "Dying well," according to Byock (2010a, 2010b), involves a political agenda that demands that more be done to help dying older adults to find relief from suffering in all contexts. Although it may require that individuals take more responsibility for their own health and well-being, it also necessitates a society that recognizes the value of family members and professionals as caregivers, and provides the necessary resources for our medical, spiritual, and educational (to name a few) institutions to actualize the morally just promotion of a good death for all.

CONCLUSION

We end this lifespan consideration of dying with a summary table (see Table 6.1) that outlines normative developmental tasks, associated concerns and issues of dying, and some pragmatic ways of handling related difficulties associated with dying. In reviewing this table, caregivers are cautioned *not* to take a "cookie-cutter" approach to their dying clients or loved ones. As Erikson (1968) so aptly noted, the developmental tasks of each age period are anticipatory and reflective of both past and future developmental needs, and thus there is considerable overlap in the issues and needs outlined in the accompanying table. What is present also is significantly influenced by individual factors (e.g., gender, race, income level), the institutional and political forces that support the dying, and cultural attitudes and belief systems that are challenged in a modern technological world. No matter what the age or developmental period, preserving dignity and fostering a sense of personal integrity in the face of dying should be a fundamental human right across the globe.

REFERENCES

Arnett, J. J. (2000). *Emerging adulthood: The winding road from the late teens through the twenties*. New York: Oxford University Press.

Avert, International HIV and AIDS Charity. (2011). *The HIV and AIDS epidemic in Africa*. Available at http://www.avert.org/aidssouthafrica.htm

Bluebond-Langner, M. (1978). *The private worlds of dying children*. Princeton, NJ: Princeton University Press.

Burnham, G., Doocy, S., Dzeng, E., Lafta, R., & Roberts, L. (2006). *The human cost of war: A mortality study 2002–2006*. Baltimore, MD: Johns Hopkins University.

Byock, I. (2010a). It is time for our generation to act courageously. *The Forum, 36*(1), 3–5.

Byock, I. (2010b). *Dying with dignity*. Hastings Center Report. Retrieved from www.dyingwithdignity.org

Capron, A. M. (2007). Legal and ethical problems in decisions for death. *The Journal of Law, Medicine & Ethics, 14*, 141–144.

Chochinov, H. M. (2006). Dying, dignity, and new horizons in palliative end-of-life care. *CA: A Cancer Journal for Clinicians, 56*, 84–103.

Cook, A. S., & Oltjenbruns, K. A. (1998). *Dying and grieving: Lifespan and family perspectives* (2nd ed.). Fort Worth, TX: Harcourt Brace.

Corr, C. A. (1992). A task-based approach to coping with dying. *Omega, Journal of Death and Dying, 24*, 81–94.

Cupit, I. N., Servaty-Seib, H. L., Parikh, S. T., Walker, A. C., & Martin, R. (under review). College and the grieving student: A mixed-methods analysis.

Demmer, C. (2009). Adolescents and HIV/AIDS. In D. E. Balk, & C. A. Corr (Eds.), *Adolescent encounters with death, bereavement, and coping* (pp. 99–114). New York: Springer Publishing.

Dickens, D. S. (2010). Comparing pediatric deaths with and without hospice support. *Pediatric Blood Cancer, 54*, 746–750.

Erikson, E. (1968). *Identity, youth, and crisis*. New York: W.W. Norton.

Feifel, H. (Ed.). (1977). *New meanings of death*. New York: McGraw-Hill.

Fishlinger, A. (2010). *Look Good . . . Feel Better Newsletter, 11*(2). Retrieved from http://lookgoodfeelbetter.org

Fowler, K., Poehling, K., Billheimer, D., Hamilton, R., Wu, H., Mulder, J. et al. (2006). Hospice referral practices for children with cancer: A survey of pediatric oncologists. *Journal of Clinical Oncology, 24*, 1099–1104.

Freyer, D. R. (2004). Care of the dying adolescent: Special considerations. *Pediatrics, 113*, 381–388.

Glaser, B., & Strauss, A. (1965). *Awareness of dying*. Chicago: Aldine.

Gostin, L. O. (2005). Ethics, the constitution, and the dying process. *Journal of the American Medical Association, 293*, 2403–2407.

Gupta, L. M. (2008, May). *Addressing traumatic losses among war-affected children in the developing world: Lessons learned for future post-conflict interventions*. Keynote address presented to the 30th Annual Conference of the Association for Death Education and Counseling, Montreal, CA.

Jones, A. L., Moss, A. J., & Harris-Kojetin, L. D. (2011) *Use of advance directives in long-term care populations*. NCHS data brief, no 54. Hyattsville, MD: National Center for Health Statistics.

Kastenbaum, R. (1972). On the future of death: Some images and options. *Omega: Journal of Death and Dying, 3*, 306–318.

Kastenbaum, R. (2004). *On our way: The final passage through life and death.* Berkeley, CA: University of California Press.

Kastenbaum, R. (2012). *Death, society, and human experience* (11th ed.). Upper Saddle River, NJ: Pearson.

Kübler-Ross, E. (1969). *On death and dying.* New York: Macmillan.

Lunney, J. R., Lynn, J., Foley, D. J., Lipson, S., & Guralnik, J. M. (2003). Patterns of functional decline at the end of life. *Journal of the American Medical Association, 289,* 2387–2392.

McClain, C. S., Rosenfeld, B., & Breitbart, W. (2003). Effects of spiritual well-being on end-of-life despair in terminally-ill patients. *Lancet, 361,* 1603–1607.

Murphy, S. L., Xu, J. Q., & Kochanek, K. D. (2012). Preliminary data for 2010. *National vital statistics reports, 60* (4). Hyattsville, MD: National Center for Health Statistics. Retrieved from http://www.cdc.gov/

National Hospice and Palliative Care Organization. (2010, September). *Facts and figures: Hospice care in America.* Alexandria, VA: Author.

Neugarten, B. L., & Datan, N. (1973). Sociological perspectives on the life cycle. In P. B. Baltes, & K. W. Schaie (Eds.), *Lifespan developmental psychology: Personality and socialization* (pp. 53–79). New York: Academic Press.

Noppe, I. C., & Noppe, L. D. (2009). Adolescents, accidents and homicides. In D. E. Balk, & C. A. Corr (Eds.), *Adolescent encounters with death, bereavement, and coping* (pp. 61–79). New York: Springer.

Roberts, B. W., Kuncel, N. R., Shiner, R., Caspi, A., & Goldberg, L. R. (2007). The power of personality: The comparative validity of personality traits, socioeconomic status, and cognitive ability for predicting important life outcomes. *Perspectives on Psychological Science, 2,* 313–345.

Romm, R. (2009). *The mercy papers. A memoir of three weeks.* New York: Scribner.

Sofka, C. J., Cupit, I. N., & Gilbert, K. R. (Eds.). (2012). *Dying, death, and grief in an online universe: For counselors and educators.* New York: Springer Publishing.

Stevens, M. M., Dunsmore, J. C., Bennett, D. L., & Young, A. J. (2009). Adolescents living with life-threatening illnesses. In D. E. Balk, & C. A. Corr (Eds.), *Adolescent encounters with death, bereavement, and coping* (pp. 115–139). New York: Springer.

UN Inter-agency Group for Child Mortality Estimation (2011, September 14). *Levels and trends in child mortality: Report 2011.* Retrieved from http://www.childinfo.org/mortality_overview.html

Walsh, M. (2010). Cancer in children and adolescents: Psychosocial dimensions. In K. J. Doka, & A. S. Tucci (Eds.), *Living with grief: Cancer and end-of-life care* (pp. 137–146). Washington, DC: Hospice Foundation of America.

Zawistowski, C. A., & DeVita, M. A. (2004). A descriptive study of children dying in the pediatric intensive care unit after withdrawal of life-sustaining treatment. *Pediatric Critical Care Medicine, 5,* 216–223.

7

Mental Health Symptom Management for Clients Who Are Near the End of Life

JACKSON P. RAINER AND JOHNATHAN C. MARTIN

Because of their influence on decision making and quality of life, mental health issues are relevant in the consideration of end-of-life care. This chapter focuses on mental health symptom identification and management. Individuals struggling with end-of-life issues who are differentially incapacitated by transient or chronic mental illness will be discussed in terms of decision making, treatment, and quality of life.

Near the end of life, emphasis is obviously placed on medical aspects of care; however, significantly less attention is paid to those psychological, psychosocial, and psychiatric concerns that are comorbid to physical problems. Certainly, although the focus of attention should be on physical need, comprehensive treatment requires that mental health deficits be assessed and addressed, as these psychological and interpersonal factors play an important role in the dying process. Particularly throughout the last two decades, the role of mental health continues to be addressed as crucial in the dying process, as evidenced in a World Health Organization (1990) policy report on end-of-life care that states "control of pain, of other symptoms, and of psychological, social, and spiritual problems is paramount in palliative care" (p. 11).

In addition to policy statements inclusive of psychological and psychosocial health management near the end of life, the research literature and clinical practice clearly direct clinicians to attend to the mental health of the patient and intimate system during care offered for terminal illnesses. Attention is to be focused on the alleviation of pain and suffering, where pain is defined as "an unpleasant sensory and emotional experience associated with actual or potential tissue damage, or described in terms of such damage" (International Association for the Study of Pain [IASP] Task Force on Taxonomy, 1994, p. 209). Research demonstrates that physical pain can lead to or exacerbate psychological pain, particularly clinical depression, and heightened anxiety (Block, 2000). Therefore, the alleviation of pain is important not only in terms of providing complete, quality care for the dying person, but also in moderating the role that corresponding mental health factors play in end-of-life decisions. The reduction of suffering can improve the quality of life of dying individuals and their caregiving and intimate support systems. Suffering has been eloquently defined as,

> ... a more expansive concept than pain. It goes beyond unpleasant sensations or distressing symptoms to encompass the anguish, terror, and hopelessness that dying patients may experience. A dying person who experiences few if any physical symptoms may suffer greatly if he or she feels that life has lost any meaning ... Subjective perceptions of suffering may have significant emotional and spiritual dimensions related to self-image, family relationships, past experience, caregiver attitudes, and other circumstances of a patient's life. (Field & Cassel, 1997, p. 26)

A female patient of one of the authors, living in advanced stages of colon cancer, described her experience with pain and suffering in this way.

CASE 1:

I have been in physical pain much of the time since I was diagnosed 2 years ago. I had surgery to resect my colon, and then chemotherapy and radiation therapy. I was advised of the risks, potential side effects, and possible benefits of treatment. I thought I was ready for whatever they could throw at me. Nobody told me, though, about how anxious I would be. I've put on a brave face, but at heart, I've always been fairly edgy. I know this to be my natural temperament. Even before I was diagnosed, I would've characterized myself as "electric." Now, I'm just anxious. Because I have limited physical energy, I spin in my thoughts much of the time. My grand ideas, creative energies, and optimistic outlook about life have given way to obsessions, misery, and worry. I try to hold on to myself, but it is getting harder. There are days that I want to crawl out of my skin.

My treatment team has given me the option of salvage therapy or palliative care. Do you know the definition of salvage? It means to "save from peril." This is not my favorite definition, even though I feel like I am in great danger. I have been hoping for a cure. I'm trying to adjust to the end of life and my coming death with as little pain as I must endure, and as much peace as I can muster. I really would like to die in character, as the creative eccentric I used to know was myself. I hate seeing myself as an anxious, fussy, worry wort. I'm embarrassed to talk about my anxiety, and my care team is even more embarrassed than I am when I bring it up. They tell me not to worry, and that everything that can be done, is being done. That is not reassuring, nor does it soothe me.

As illustrated in this example, end-of-life concerns are likely to change an individual's sense of self. The figure/ground of the physical illness and its emotional correlates create a dynamic process for coping with impending death. Mental health needs, such as anxiety and depression, are often ignored or shunted to the side. Doka (1996, p. 116) commented on the figural task of holding the mental health and quality of life of the dying person. He said:

> Life-threatening illness is only part of life. Throughout the time of the illness ... individuals continue to meet many needs and to cope with all the issues and problems that they had prior to the diagnosis ... [Of course,] the experience of illness may affect the perception of these needs and issues ... All the previous challenges of life—dealing with family and friends, coping with work and finances, even keeping up with the demands of a home or apartment—remain an ongoing part of the larger struggle of life and living.

Because research and clinical practice have documented that the mental health of an individual can have significant impact on quality of life and end-of-life decision making, these matters should be at the forefront when providing services to those who are dying. However, this is rarely the case. Unnoticed or unmanaged symptoms can precipitate a crisis that could have been prevented or addressed from a more proactive perspective.

DECISION MAKING AND DIAGNOSIS

Mental health symptom presentation during end-of-life care requires careful thought to prioritize issues and concerns for the client, caregiver, and intimate system. The clinician's critical thinking should raise vital questions and then clearly and precisely formulate treatment trajectories for defined problems. The key task revolves around gathering and assessing figural information to arrive at well-reasoned conclusions and solutions that can be tested against relevant criteria, standards, and research. Therefore, a formal assessment is necessary to evaluate and articulate a reasonable treatment plan. Assessment is defined as a time-limited, crystallized process that collects clinical information from many sources in order to reach a diagnosis, make a prognosis, render a biopsychosocial formulation, and to determine treatment (Maxmen & Ward, 1995). A thorough assessment contains relevant history, the client's mental status, principal complaints, and contextual findings in regard to disease state.

Diagnostic formulations define clinical entities and syndromes so that clinicians have the same understanding of what the diagnostic category means, as defined by the *Diagnostic and Statistical Manual of Mental Disorders IV*'s (*DSM-IV*; American Psychiatric Association [APA], 2000) rubric for an atheoretical multiaxial description of symptoms and circumstances. A disorder is marked by benchmark cardinal symptoms, with a natural history, etiology, and pathogenesis. The purpose of diagnosis is to determine treatment. In the age of efficacy-based interventions and best practices, the diagnosis provides a valid, reliable, and scientifically sound beginning point that informs treatment options.

According to *DSM*, nosology, psychopathology and the manifestation of mental disorders must produce clinically significant impairment in an individual's personal, social, or occupational life; biological changes may or may not be involved. Pathology manifests as symptoms, distress, and disability. The disability can be directly observed and documented objectively; however, symptoms are experienced subjectively, cannot always be observed, and must be reported by the client. The challenge for the practitioner lies in determining whether the presentation of symptoms is pathological or developmental (e.g., related to the end-of-life period) in nature (see Exhibit 7.1).

The clinician should examine multiple rubrics for explaining an individual's phenomenological experience. In the example above, the client could easily be diagnosed with an anxiety disorder. However, her distress could also be understood as an authentic and congruent frame of reference in relation to a diminished set of effective coping skills and strategies. In addition to considering symptoms as pathology, Rando (1993) suggested three major psychological and behavioral patterns that emerge near the end of life. They include (1) retreat and conservation of energy, (2) exclusion from the threat of death, and (3) attempts to master or control the threat of death. Using this rubric, the client's anxiety may be viewed as a change of energy and focus.

The caution for clinicians is related to over-diagnosis. Differential diagnosis is the process of choosing the correct diagnosis from conditions

EXHIBIT 7.1

Mental Health Diagnosis at End-of-Life

Although pathology can certainly exist on its own, it is more likely that mental health issues will emerge in conjunction with the disease. Before engaging in a full multiaxial assessment that searches for psychopathology, the clinician can engage in a more benign review, based on the following question:

- Are there extremes of emotions that seem foreign to the individual and can be objectively observed by others?
- Is the presentation of the syndrome of behavior affect a long-standing personality pattern, or is it new to the individual?

with similar features. A general question should be initially considered: Is the individual's condition caused by a known condition or drug? If not, then the issue, according to *DSM* nosology, is determining whether there is ego-dystonic impairment of functioning. For the woman in the example, much of her anxiety seems reasonable, based on the stress associated with treatment trajectories. In her view, however, the toxicity of the anxiety feels progressively foreign to her understanding of self and becomes limiting of her capacity to be fully involved with activities of daily living. As a general rule, the clinician can avoid over-diagnosing by determining the overall and distinctive features of the presenting complaint.

Depending on the clinician's findings, essential treatment proceeds in the least intrusive way. There are any number of diagnosable mental disorders and conditions that can be addressed in order to alleviate the suffering of a dying person and maximize the quality of remaining life. Although a complete discussion of all possible disorders is beyond the scope of this chapter, the most common, debilitating, and ameliorable ones are examined (see also Chochinov & Breitbart, 2000).

ANXIETY DISORDERS

Overview

In 2010, anxiety disorders (classified according to *DSM-IV* criteria) accounted for the most common class of psychological disorders among citizens of the United States. In the general population, there is a lifetime prevalence rate of 28.8% and a 12-month prevalence rate of 18.1% for anxiety disorders affecting individuals at a given time (Kessler, Chiu, Demler, & Walters, 2005). In the context of this chapter, it is important to consider prevalence to the degree that individuals are impacted by anxiety disorders near the end of life.

Elder care should be particularly considered. As of 2000, approximately 35 million U.S. residents were aged 65 or older, with a projection that this number will double by the year 2030 (McGuire, 2009). Recent studies indicate that the prevalence of anxiety disorders increases in older adults when lower education, single marital status, and disability are taken into account (Gum, King-Kallimanis, & Kohn, 2009). For the mental health practitioner, these dynamics bring strong potential impact for treating anxiety disorders in patients near the end of life.

Although anxiety disorders are among the most treatable disorders, only approximately one-third of sufferers seek treatment (Anxiety Disorders Association of America [ADAA], 2011). For patients near the end of life, this may occur for a variety of reasons, such as cost of treatment, geographic disadvantages, limited mobility, and lack of recognition that the anxiety may be treatable (Newman, Szkody, Llera, & Przeworski, 2011). According to the ADAA (2011), additional hindrances to treatment stem from older patients' tendencies to report physical complaints rather than psychiatric symptoms. For these reasons, diagnostic and treatment efforts become complicated because of the underrecognition of symptomatological underpinnings. Therefore, increasing recognition of the more common anxiety-related symptoms is paramount. "Normal" anxiety serves as a natural response to stimuli that are perceived as threatening to one's well-being. However, when these natural responses become excessive, they become debilitating and unhealthy.

Diagnostic Implications

Conceptualized as a multidimensional construct, anxiety has been described as a system consisting of three parts: subjective distress, physiological response, and avoidance behavior (Beidel, Turner, & Alfano, 2003). In respect to the treatment of anxiety for end-of-life patients, a model is suggested to practitioners, constructed of three categories of anxiety (Foti, 2003). These categories consist of (1) reactive anxiety, (2) symptomatic anxiety, and (3) previous anxiety. As the name implies, reactive anxiety is the patient's response to the distress and disability surrounding illness and treatment, as well as states of intense emotion that impair functioning (e.g., fear of the dying process) and often result in a patient's lack of desire or willingness to comply with treatment protocols. Symptomatic anxiety refers to the agitation and "out of control" feelings that emerge in the presence of intense physical pain associated with the illness or withdrawal from medications. The third category, previous anxiety, may reflect the patient's history of past anxiety experiences, which can be exacerbated as the patient's sense of control over situational factors diminishes. Thorough assessment addressing each of these areas is necessary for obtaining a clear diagnostic picture, which is vital for determining appropriate treatment strategies.

Treatment

Because of the special nature of end-of-life treatment, longer-term psychotherapy may be better suited for the patient's family and loved ones who experience anxiety either during or after the patient's death. As discussed later in this chapter, family members who feel unprepared for the death of a loved one generally experience greater anxiety (Herbert, Schulz, Copeland, & Arnold, 2009). For the terminally ill patient, brief interventions oriented toward symptom reduction are likely to be more amenable approaches to treatment. For example, simply providing information about diagnosis and the dying process may help to alleviate some of the patient's reactive distress associated with the illness (Werth, Gordon, & Johnson, 2002). The management of physical pain is especially important because increased pain tends to exacerbate psychological distress (Foti, 2003). Finally, cognitive and behavioral approaches have been shown to be important adjuncts not only in pain management, but also in soothing the impact of the dying process for both patient and family. Other specific recommendations for mental health practitioners include (1) acting as an intermediary for communication between physician and patient/family, (2) advocating for a client-centered model of care, (3) focusing on the quality of remaining life, and (4) implementing discussions of the dying process earlier in the patient's care (Larson & Tobin, 2000).

By increasing the recognition of anxiety-related symptoms, facilitating the provision of information surrounding the dying process, and advocating for better communication between patient and physician, mental health practitioners serve as important conduits for the diagnosis and treatment of anxiety-related disorders near the end of life.

MOOD DISORDERS

Overview

In addition to anxiety disorders, mood disorders comprise one of the most common categories of mental health problems. Major debilitating effects of mood disorders parallel those of the impact of heart disease on one's quality of life (Areán & Chatav, 2003). According to the National Institute of Mental Health (NIMH, 2008a), mood disorders have a lifetime prevalence rate of 20.8%, and a 12-month prevalence rate of 9.5% at any given time for adults in the United States. To aid in conceptualization, mood disorders can be dichotomized into related, but distinct, groups: (1) depressive disorders and (2) bipolar disorders.

The first group, Depressive Disorders, consists of Major Depressive Disorder, Dysthymic/disorder, and Depressive Disorder Not Otherwise Specified (APA, 2000). Consistent with *DSM* nosology, all three types share similar features: mood symptoms, vegetative symptoms, and cognitive symptoms (Areán & Chatav, 2003). Major Depressive Disorder, as a category, has a lifetime prevalence rate of 16.5% in adults and a 12-month prevalence rate of 6.7% in the general population at any given time (NIMH, 2008b). Although Dysthymia is a much more persistent disorder, lasting at least 2 years, lifetime and 12-month prevalence rates among adults are much lower at 2.5% and 1.5%, respectively (NIMH, 2008c).

The second of the two groups, Bipolar Disorders, comprises Bipolar I and Bipolar II Disorders, Cyclothymic Disorder, and Bipolar Disorder Not Otherwise Specified (APA, 2000). Often referred to by their colloquial name of "manic-depression," Bipolar Disorders are conceptualized as extreme shifts in mood along a continuum between two poles (i.e., depression and mania). On one end of the continuum, Bipolar I Disorder is generally characterized with a greater frequency of manic and mixed episodes (that may or may not include psychotic features), while Bipolar II is commonly distinguished by multiple depressive episodes (on the opposite end of the continuum), with occasional interruption of a hypomanic episode (Lohr & Cook, 2003). Like Bipolar Disorders I and II, Cyclothymia is marked by mood fluctuations along the continuum between depression and mania. These fluctuations are generally less extreme, with both hypomanic and depressive symptoms/episodes occurring more frequently than in Bipolar I and II Disorders (APA, 2000). All Mood Disorders, including Bipolar Disorders, can cause severe dysfunction in personal, social, and occupational areas of life. Approximately 3.9% of adult Americans will be affected by a mood disorder at any given time (NIMH, 2008a). Subsyndromal depressions (e.g., Dysthymia and Minor Depression) affect as many as 20% of the elderly population in particular (Areán & Chatav, 2003).

Diagnostic Implications

Mental health practitioners faced with the differential diagnosis of depressive disorders in the general population must consider a variety of factors such as medical illness, drug and alcohol abuse, grief and bereavement, and depressive symptoms because of other psychiatric disorders. Research continues to show that health-related and developmental issues (e.g., chronic illness, widowhood) associated with later life will often trigger depressive symptoms (Mental Health America [MHA], 2011). Therefore, diagnostic implications for the terminally ill may require special attention and acute awareness of both the patient's medical illness and the potential bereavement issues surrounding personal experience near the end of life. These variables are prone to exacerbate depressive symptoms. As such, authors remind clinicians that subtle variations in patients' presentations should be accounted for when differentiating between diagnoses. For example, Werth, Gordon, and Johnson (2002) note that an endogenous clinical depression is a less common feature in the dying process. This type of distinction between major depressive disorder and a situation-oriented depression would indicate modifications of the standard treatment approach for a major depressive disorder.

Though the proper assessment of depression will involve observation and use of self-report measures during the clinical interview, near the end of life, the most common means of assessment is subjective report. Regarding instrumentation, rapid assessment inventories such as the Beck Depression Inventory-II (BDI-II) and the Center for Epidemiological Studies-Depression Scale (CES-D), and the Primary Care Evaluation of Mental Disorders

(PRIME-MD) identify "red flags" for depression that warrant further inquiry on the part of the clinician (Areán & Chatav, 2003). Best practice guidelines suggest that regular assessment is equally as important as accurate assessment.

In respect to medical illness, increased depressive symptoms also appear to be associated with self-harm behavior (e.g., withdrawing from treatment) for patients suffering from terminal illnesses (McDade-Montez, Christensen, Cvengros, & Lawton, 2006). Because of the risk of self-harm, regular suicide assessment is paramount for practitioners working with older adults, especially considering that the risk of suicidal ideation increases with age, with Caucasian men older than 65 carrying the highest rates of suicide deaths (Meeks, Vahia, Lavretsky, Kulkarni, & Jeste, 2011). In other recent studies, the instability of symptom presentation and causal factors of depression (among others) in end-of-life patients suggests that practitioners must be keenly attuned to such variations (Hayduk, Olson, Quan, Cree, & Cui, 2010). An in-depth discussion of suicide and self-harm is beyond the scope of this chapter, though it remains a worthy consideration for the clinician (see Exhibit 7.2).

Treatment

Because older adults and terminally ill patients endorse physical complaints, practitioners must be prepared to translate these reports into observable behavioral symptomatology. For example, where patients might describe sleep disturbance and lethargy, clinicians should look to corresponding psychological components such as flat affect, tearfulness, social withdrawal, pessimism, and decreased reactivity (Endicott, 1984). For the patient near the

---

EXHIBIT 7.2

Assessing Self-Harm and Suicidality

- Observe and assess pain, depression, and delirium
- Isolation, abandonment, and unmanaged pain increase the affective sense of hopelessness, which increases the likelihood for depression
- Delirious patients are more likely to be impulsive
- Assess mental status continuously, particularly in terms of the patient's understanding of the illness and presenting symptoms
- Assess vulnerability factors and pain control
- Assess the support system and all external controls

Remember: Suicidality increases if there is a premorbid history of a psychological disorder.

end of life, these components become the focus of treatment. One treatment model, proposed by Young, Beck, and Weinberger (1993), outlined a rubric for conceptualizing depression where cognitive, behavioral, and affective variables are interrelated. Other work has found that the person's self-appraisals (cognitive), attempts to problem solve (behavior), and successful reduction of symptoms (affect), appear to correspond in an interactive fashion (Areán & Chatav, 2003).

There is little contemporary information available that speaks specifically to the treatment of subclinical depressions in older adults. However, tailoring treatments integrating behavior therapy, cognitive–behavioral therapy, and reminiscence/narrative therapy to the patient's needs has shown promise (Meeks et al., 2011). Though the identification of cognitive distortions and negative automatic thoughts are important for gaining a clearer understanding of the maintaining factors of depression for clients in general, this may be erroneous when working with the terminally ill if true physical symptoms (e.g., pain resulting from illness) are not addressed at the onset of the depression. Researchers point out that one of the most common debilitating cognitions of the depressed person is the hopeless view of the future (Young et al., 1993). For the terminally ill patient, however, this perspective may be a reality rather than a distorted cognition. Akin to the treatment of anxiety, clinicians initially serve as a sounding board and advocate for the depressed patient and family in their realization and integration of the ultimate outcome of illness. In this capacity, discussion about death can reduce symptoms and paradoxically increase the patient's quality of life.

To further aid in this process, contemporary mental health practitioners have begun to recognize the importance of exploration and investigation of issues surrounding religion and spirituality (Jotkowitz, Clarfield, & Glick, 2005). There is little surprise that this significant piece of human existence has received little attention in the medical literature over the years. On the basis of clinical experience of the authors, however, it is believed that by facilitating dialogue about one's spiritual domain as it relates to personal existence, practitioners can afford clients a safe place to experience meaning making, and ultimately receive a more genuine sense of peace.

DELIRIUM

Overview

Delirium is a common and distressing symptom that constitutes a significant challenge for end-of-life care. Delirium arises from a variety of causes. Drug effects are the most common. Hypnotics, narcotics, steroids, chemotherapy, and infection control agents all hold the potential to alter sensorium. Near the end of life, physical changes in the natural decline of the individual may also lead to delirium. Such changes are the result of organ failure, metabolic changes (e.g., thyroid or adrenal failure), electrolyte imbalance, infection, and nutritional state.

There are reliable techniques for the diagnosis and effective treatment of delirium. According to the *DSM-IV*, delirium is characterized by a disturbance of consciousness, cognition, and perception, with a wave-like course that may fluctuate over a period of hours (APA, 2000). Delirium occurs in 28% to 83% of patients near the end of life, depending on the population studied and the criteria used (Pereira, Hanson, & Bruera, 1997). Delirium is challenging because it frightens patients and their families. The presence of delirium can cause as much distress as physical pain. It is troubling to families and members of the intimate system because it limits effective communication with the patient, robbing all involved of valuable time and opportunities to make final choices and plans. For many patients, delirium is a predictor of approaching death. The overarching task for the clinician who encounters delirium is to acknowledge, facilitate, and enhance the leave-taking process for the patient and family. In general, it is a time to begin saying good-bye.

Diagnostic Implications

Often, delirium is obvious, but up to half of all episodes go unnoticed by clinicians (Francis, Strong, Martin, & Kapoor, 1988). Delirium can be easily missed because the constellation of features that define it are not readily apparent, including acute onset, inattention, altered levels of consciousness, and cognitive impairment. To diagnose, the clinician must know the individual's baseline status. Clinical skills are employed: The patient will appear disorganized, sleep–wake cycles are disturbed, the individual will be disoriented and will likely experience perceptual disturbance (e.g., illusions), there will be difficulty maintaining/shifting attention, and there will be a waxing and waning level of consciousness. The professional must make a bedside assessment of the dimensions of cognitive impairment and deficits of attention. Many clinicians prefer to use the more formal Mini-Mental State Examination to assess cognition (Folstein, Folstein, & McHugh, 1975). Administration is quick and easy, though this instrument does not distinguish between dementia and delirium. An alternative assessment tool is the Memorial Delirium Assessment Scale, which correlates well with other cognitive tests and can be used reliably with medically ill individuals (Breitbart, 1997) (see Exhibit 7.3).

Treatment

The decision to intervene depends on the degree to which the delirium is distressing. Intervention strategies can be made independently and

EXHIBIT 7.3

Don't Confuse Delirium With Dementia

Delirium	Dementia
Onset is rapid	Onset is progressive
Symptoms have a fluctuating level and severity	Symptoms are consistent, progressive, and worsening
Reversible	Irreversible
Less memory impairment	More memory impairment
Emergency	Nonemergent

concurrently to the search for a cause. The course of delirium is highly variable. Clinicians will need to remain alert to the possibility of immediate development and/or escalating presentation of distressing symptoms.

Pharmacological treatment is the preferred "front line" intervention for addressing symptoms of delirium. The goal of medication management is to help the patient return as closely to baseline as is possible, without sedation. Concurrent counseling interventions should be directed to reality orientation and reinforcement of adaptive skills. Family interventions are also warranted, with goals directed toward education, reassurance, and support.

PERSONALITY DISORDERS

Overview

Personality traits are ingrained, enduring patterns of behaving, feeling, perceiving, and thinking that are prominent in a wide range of personal and social contexts, including the end of life (Cloninger, 2008). Personality features may or may not be adaptive. These traits become Personality Disorders when they become inflexible, maladaptive, significantly impair social and occupational functioning, or cause substantial subjective distress. Personality Disorders are longstanding. Individuals with Personality Disorders typically justify and rationalize their behavior.

Diagnostic Implications

The diagnosis of a Personality Disorder in an individual near the end of life is essentially irrelevant. The first author has often said that "People live and die in character." In general, there is little wisdom or utility in diagnosing a Personality Disorder during the dying process. A Personality Disorder diagnosis should not be made in the midst of end-of-life care without a reason for pursuing the full historical knowledge of the premorbid functioning of the individual.

Most Personality Disorders become apparent during adolescence and persist through life. Although traditional theory says they become less obvious by middle or old age (Maxmen & Ward, 1995), Personality Disorders become more pronounced during stressful circumstances, including the demands of the end of life. The *DSM* nosology divides Personality Disorders into three clusters. The first consists of Paranoid, Schizoid, and Schizotypal Personality Disorders, characterized by odd or eccentric behavior. The second includes Histrionic, Narcissistic, Antisocial, and Borderline Personality Disorders, characterized by dramatic, overemotional, and erratic behavior. The third cluster consists of Avoidant, Dependent, and Obsessive–Compulsive Personality Disorders, characterized by highly anxious and fearful affects.

Treatment

The influence of personality characteristics and how individuals cope with various challenges near the end of life has not been extensively studied. However, because individuals with Personality Disorders can be disruptive to care efforts, discussion of treatment is warranted. Much of the available data on Personality Disorders near the end of life relies on the psychoanalytic term *neuroticism* rather than using *DSM* observational descriptions to distinguish the depth of pathology present (Chochinov et al., 2006). In general psychodynamic terms, neurotic behavior is subjectively experienced by an individual as uncharacteristic of the usual "self" (i.e., as being significantly different). In contrast, the pathological behavior exhibited by an individual with a Personality Disorder is congruent, customary, and predictable within an individual, subjective frame of reference. Neurotic behavior can develop at any time and is seen as defensive and protective. When threatened or under stress (e.g., near the end of life), personality pathology becomes more pronounced, though this is almost always unrecognized by the patient exhibiting the symptoms. However, others are usually uncomfortable with their "neurotic" behavior. Personality Disorders are longstanding and in character with the individual's understanding of self, no matter how problematic or distressing the behavior may be to others.

Individuals are prone to exhibit more ego-dystonic behavior and affect near the end of life. Sources of distress include depression, anxiety, sense of dignity, quality of life, autonomy, hopelessness, concentration, and outlook for the future. These associations are expressed across the psychological, existential, and, to a lesser extent, physical and social domains of end-of-life distress (Chochinov et al., 2006). Individuals who have more pronounced pathology defined by the manifestation of the Personality Disorder will have even poorer adjustment to the demands of end-of-life trajectories and care. Essentially, the greater the pathology, the less likely the individual will be to find a wellspring of coping skills to meet the demands of the end of life.

Difficult Personality Disorders or interpersonal styles can significantly affect the responsiveness of professional and intimate caregivers. It is not unusual to experience a bias of professional judgment, assessment, or treatment planning for individuals with Personality Disorders (Block & Billings, 1998). Because the individual with a Personality Disorder is inflexible and increasingly brittle in the presence of ongoing stress, clinicians will need to address systemic concerns. It is common that any decision made for the individual may be unsatisfactory. Issues related to autonomy/control, dignity, and fear will be clouded by the problematic behavior of the individual. Interventions must be made on behalf of, rather than in concert with, the patient. Clinicians should be alert to caregiver compassion fatigue and attentive to countertransference. Individuals living with a Personality Disorder near the end of life can be challenging, frustrating, and maddening. The treatment team should be aware of their own beliefs and unresolved issues and conflicts, as they may significantly affect treatment decisions.

TRAUMA

Overview

Providers of clinical services may potentially act as medical triage team members. Therefore, mental health professionals should be aware of trauma and its impact on individuals in order to practice competently and ethically. It comes as no surprise that trauma work is commonplace for mental health clinicians. In fact, the results of a recent survey of clinical psychologists reported an average of 14.3 practice hours per month spent working with survivors of trauma (Cook, Dinnen, Rehman, Bufka, & Courtois, 2011). Despite its impact on the psyche, and in contrast to disorders with similar prevalence rates, trauma has received an insufficient amount of attention from researchers until the past few decades. Before the formal diagnostic criteria were established for post-traumatic stress disorder (PTSD), which came into being with the *DSM-III*, the effects of trauma were labeled by more passive names, such as "transient situational disturbance" (Calhoun & Resick, 1993). Fortunately, the gaps of information on "trauma psychology" are now being investigated with more fervor, particularly since the inception of the American Psychological Association's most recent addition, Division 56 (Division of Trauma Psychology, 2010). As more research is conducted, clinicians practice within their scope of competence through familiarity with the basic conceptualization of trauma and current practice standards.

The event of trauma is unique. It is differentiated from other disorders based on a number of factors such as the rapidity of onset, frequency and intensity of traumatic experiences, and the amount of time the individual requires for the characteristic hyperaroused state to return to baseline once activated by internal or environmental experience (Jaffe, Segal, & Dumke, 2005). Traumatic experiences can be derived from a seemingly endless list of possibilities, with onset resulting from either physical or emotional injury, or more often, both. The impact of trauma affects a sobering proportion of citizens in the United States. For example, in 2008, hospital-based emergency departments in the United States reported more than 123,000,000 visits, with approximately 46,700,000—nearly one-third—of these being admitted to emergency department trauma centers. Overall, triage teams classified 38.9% of these visits as "urgent," 11.9% as "emergent," and 3.7% as "immediate" in respect to their degree of psychological severity at presentation (Centers for Disease Control and Prevention [CDC], 2008). Consideration, then, must also be given to the families of sufferers whose lives are impacted as well. With the U.S. Census Bureau's (2009) estimated average family size of 3.19 members, it could be assumed that the number of immediate family members directly impacted by trauma are more than triple the above estimates. End-of-life issues and concerns may certainly be considered as activating events for trauma response for a terminally ill person or members of the intimate system.

Diagnostic Implications

Because trauma is a subsequent effect to immediate and unforeseen events, it is difficult to draw clear distinctions about how an individual may react. More specifically, an experience of trauma is linked more closely to an individual's perception of an event rather than to the event itself. For example, although one individual may experience nightmares and hypervigilance in the weeks and months following a horrendous motor vehicle collision, a second individual involved in the same event may experience none of these posttraumatic symptoms. Because everyone reacts differently to crisis situations, clinicians are directed to the diagnostic literature to begin forming hypotheses for individual clients. Primarily, practitioners should initially look for two key components: (1) an experience of witnessing actual or threatened death or serious injury, and (2) a response to the first component that involves intense fear, helplessness, or horror (APA, 2000).

These criteria provide a solid foundation for conducting appropriate assessment. For individuals and families near the end of life, this is a crucial element for best practice, especially because it has been revealed in the research literature that crisis intervention has the potential to do more harm than good when implemented with persons who would otherwise be able to cope relatively independent of outside resources (Brock, n.d.). On the other hand, physical trauma can leave victims incapacitated to the point that they are unable to express their desires. When this is the case, such as end-of-life circumstances for individuals suffering cognitive dysfunction (e.g., closed head injury or where the victim resides in a vegetative state), family members may find themselves in a state of heightened vulnerability and emotional volatility. Before any form of treatment can begin, clinicians must make it their priority to ensure the safety of all those involved. As such, assessing for trauma near the end of life is equally or perhaps even more relevant for family members of the dying person.

Treatment

Trauma requires treating both the dying patient and family members (Rainer & Brown, 2007). Processing and meaning making of associated feelings about the dying experience, for the patient, caregiver, or family member, can prove beneficial. The degree of coping flexibility espoused by each individual will differ and emotional reactivity is not uncommon. The clinician's approach to treatment not only hinges on the immediate impact of potential death or injury, but also on the patient's and family members' tried and true coping strategies. A solution-focused approach (Rainer & Brown, 2007) to help trauma survivors and their families move past the event may be necessary before an existential, meaning-making therapeutic process can begin. Identifying and teaching basic distress tolerance skills (e.g., diaphragmatic breathing, progressive muscle relaxation, and visual imagery) to both patients and their loved ones may prove useful in the face of more immediate threats. For the dying patient, such skills may help to alleviate some of the distress perpetuated by the feeling of loss of control. For the family members, encouraging and facilitating effective and adaptive functioning during a time of crisis is crucial when many life and death decisions must be made with little or no opportunity for considering their potential consequences.

CASE 2:

An elderly patriarch was brought to the emergency department following a heart attack. Once stabilized, he was moved to a hospital room with his family in attendance. It had been determined that the man had no advance directives and was at the point of death. Medical personnel contacted the counselor when the family appeared immobilized and unable to make effective decisions about how to provide end-of-life care. The counselor interviewed the family. The oldest adult daughter said, "My dad has been an abusive alcoholic for years. He did all of his dirty work behind closed doors. I've waited for years to see him this helpless. Now that I see him, it isn't at all like I imagined. None of us know what to do. I still don't feel safe. We are tied in a knot."

A word of caution is warranted for practitioners who spend significant amounts of time providing clinical services to trauma victims and survivors. It is of no coincidence that the topic of caregiver burnout receives ample attention by researchers in medical, mental health, and social work professions. Despite best efforts to maintain a sense of professional and emotional distance from the vast amounts of pain seen in the line of duty, mental health professionals cannot walk away unaffected, particularly in the presence of trauma. Over time, this can become a critical ethical issue. In the Winter 2010 newsletter of the American Psychological Association's Trauma Psychology Division (American Psychological Association Division 56, 2010), practitioners were reminded that the human capacity to employ genuine sensitivity to clients is limited; moreover, this capacity tends to decrease as the amount of losses reaches catastrophic levels. With this is mind, clinicians must engage in continual and consistent self-evaluation throughout trauma work to ensure that the ethical principles of nonmaleficence and beneficence are sufficiently incorporated into treatment.

SUBSTANCE ABUSE AND DEPENDENCE

Overview

In light of the end-of-life demands for pain management, diagnosing addictive disease may seem like a futile endeavor. However, for substance-dependent individuals, characteristics of the disorder complicate and compromise end-of-life care in important ways. As discussed earlier in this chapter, most terminal illnesses are characterized by pain. Effective management of pain is a benchmark of best practice for the treatment team. Acknowledging and determining that patients and family members understand the meaning of the terms tolerance and physical and psychological dependence (addiction), then determining how the concerns of the system affect prescribing, dispensing, or administering medications is challenging. Recognizing the difficulties inherent in identifying addictive diseases for patients in whom opioids are therapeutically prescribed, a consensus statement was developed by the American Academy of Pain Medicine, the American Pain Society, and the American Society of Addiction Medicine in 2001. This statement provides definitions for addiction in chronic pain populations and may be extrapolated for use in end-of-life care. Addiction is defined in this public policy statement as "a primary, chronic, neurological disease, with genetic, psychosocial, and environmental factors influencing its development and manifestations" and is "characterized by behaviors that include one or more of the following: impaired control over drug use, compulsive use, continued use despite harm, and craving" (p. 8).

Diagnostic Implications

In the context of end-of-life care, addiction can be determined by the presence of certain observable patient behaviors. In the recent past, pain management has been approached with great caution, lest the patient "become addicted" to the medications that provide comfort and enhance quality near the end of life. For the clinician, this is irrelevant because pain must be well managed. However, a historical assessment of the individual's substance use history has great clinical utility, one often overlooked by the treatment team and not often or well disclosed by members of the intimate system. Addiction is defined by a craving for a drug for euphoria, by drug seeking in the absence of physical discomfort, and by manipulation of the prescriber to obtain drugs (APA, 2000). Many addicted individuals near the end of life have an inability to adhere to a prescription schedule, prefer certain forms or routes of medication, or are resistant to nonopioid treatments. Substance dependence factors into treatment planning in significant ways, including unexplained evidence of deterioration of functioning, inconsistent response to dosing regimens, drug seeking, craving and preoccupation with medication use, a preference for medications with high reward value, and poor tolerance for nonopioid and nonpharmacological treatments (see Exhibit 7.4).

CASE 3:

A 67-year-old man was admitted to an acute care unit of a rural hospital following a small stroke, complicated by an untreated kidney infection. He was diagnosed with multiple system failures. As the family gathered, the man's son-in-law met the nurse manager. "I'm doing this at great risk of my family's collective anger, but there is something you need to know: My father-in-law is an alcoholic and has been drinking daily to intoxication for over 30 years. He does have osteoarthritis, and tells us he only drinks to help his pain, but he's never seen a physician for any type of medical help. He just likes to get drunk, and he is a mean man when he gets 'likkered up,' as his wife describes him. He drinks at home, after work, and alone. He never had legal trouble... a good deal of family trouble, but nothing outside the home. We think he probably had the stroke several days ago and detoxed himself before coming to the hospital, which may be the cause of the kidney infection. His alcoholism has been a family secret for years. If we're right, he may be experiencing DTs soon, which would only make matters worse."

EXHIBIT 7.4

Is It Pain or Addiction?

Look for behavioral markers that may be indicative of drug addiction. Although no one symptom in isolation from this list should be used to diagnose a substance abuse problem, higher numbers of observed symptoms suggest and indicate the need of a more thorough substance abuse assessment. The total pattern of behavior and current and past history is necessary to make the diagnosis of substance abuse. Behavioral markers near the end of life include:

- Body language, including facial grimacing
- Clock watching
- Demanding behavior related to drug administration
- Being overly sedated after friends or family visits
- Drug paraphernalia found in the individual's environment (e.g., liquor bottles, used syringes)
- Asking for or demanding specific drugs
- Report of "drug allergies" to many opioids, but not all in the same class
- Admitting to living in an environment where family/friends are actively using drugs.

Treatment

Clinical studies demonstrate that individuals near the end of life who receive narcotics for the treatment of pain, administered and monitored by experienced practitioners, do not become addicted. Hospice experience bears this out. However, a more troubling phenomenon may be present in certain medical settings. A syndrome may arise when a patient's pain is continually undertreated and the individual begins drug seeking to obtain relief. This "pseudo-addiction" superficially resembles addictive behavior, but has two distinguishing features: The patient is in pain, and the drug-seeking behavior does not reflect individual history of substance abuse.

For the patient, treatment of pain is primary. Medical practitioners will weigh the benefits of treatment with the negative consequences associated with their unwanted side effects. For individuals near the end of life, fears of addiction or abuse are unrealistic and should not compromise pain relief decisions. Dying patients receive narcotics to relieve pain and other symptoms, not to achieve a drug-induced "high." This has been such a contentious issue that it was addressed by the United States Supreme Court in the 1990s.

Although the court did not support either using drugs to terminate life or the legitimization of drugs and controlled substances, it fully encouraged and supported adequate pain and symptom management, stating, "... A Court majority effectively requires all states to ensure that their laws do not obstruct the provision of adequate palliative care, especially for the alleviation of pain and other physical symptoms of people facing death" (Burt, 1997, p. 1234).

For the family and caregiving system, education and support are needed when the patient is a known substance abuser. Particularly when the issue is a family secret, clinicians should ensure that the treatment team is fully informed of the substance use history and current manifestations. Interventions should be prescribed to prevent further illicit substance use, including the potential for hoarding medications, or of use of more medicine than has been prescribed. Families may benefit from referrals to 12-step family groups, such as Al-Anon or Nar-Anon, for self-help during the stress of end-of-life care.

ROLE OF THE CLINICIAN: EASING THE END OF LIFE

Traditional medical care treats to cure. Near the end of life, where hopes for cure have been abandoned, patients may endure great distress. The psychosocial implications of end-of-life concerns are likely to be exacerbated by those with a mental health issue, such as anxiety and mood disorders, somatic distress, and several forms of cognitive impairment.

Communicating directly and concretely about death and dying among all parties is primary, but is oftentimes a neglected process. All communication and sharing of knowledge and expectations affects preparedness and uncertainty. Ongoing conversations identify the psychological, psychosocial, spiritual, and socioeconomic contexts of the patient and family, enabling appropriate, congruent decision making consistent with the systems' values and morals.

Thus, although they are not perfect, the best and most effective intervention for the professional to facilitate is to ensure that advance directives are in place for the patient (Rainer & McMurry, 2002). Advance directives are more fully discussed in other chapters of this book. It is worthy to restate, however, that advance directives give the patient and family choices and continued control as the disease progresses toward the end of life. A living will can give the medical team directions about the use of life-support equipment or other extraordinary means to sustain life. A second document, the health care power-of-attorney, designates a caregiver who acts as a health care proxy for the patient to make decisions when the patient is no longer able. The third advance directive is a "Do Not Resuscitate" (DNR) order, which conveys a physician's orders that a dying individual should not receive cardiopulmonary resuscitation if the patient stops breathing and/or the heart stops beating. All advance directives to the health care team give specific instructions related to end-of-life care and should be easily accessible. The documents maintain the dying individual's choice and dignity, and give caregivers the "lay of the land" regarding the dying person's wishes (Rainer & McMurry, 2002).

A terminal illness in its final stages accompanies every move within the individual's experience and casts a constant pall over the thoughts and actions of all involved. Under the best of circumstances, the experience of the end of life requires a reformulation of the self and of the system, where the pursuit of comfort takes precedence (Rainer & McMurry, 2002). In order to be helpful, practitioners must develop as much of an alliance as possible, provide reliable information related to the uncertainty of the end of life, and allow time to process information and complete important tasks.

REFERENCES

American Academy of Pain Medicine, American Pain Society, & American Society of Addiction Medicine. (2001). *Definitions related to the use of opioids for the treatment of pain: Policy statement*. Glenview, IL: Authors.

American Psychiatric Association (APA). (2000). *Diagnostic and statistical manual of mental disorders* (Revised 4th ed.), Washington, DC: American Psychiatric Press.

American Psychological Association—Division 56. (Winter, 2010). *Trauma Psychology newsletter*. Available from http://www.apatraumadivision.org/publications/newsletter_2010_fallwinter.pdf.

Anxiety Disorders Association of America. (2011). *Understanding anxiety: Facts and statistics*. Available at http://www.adaa.org/about-adaa/press-room/facts-statistics

Areán, P. A., & Chatav, Y. (2003). Mood disorders: Depressive disorders. In M. Hersen, & S. M. Turner (Eds.), *Adult psychopathology and diagnosis* (4th ed.) (pp. 286–312). Hoboken, NJ: John Wiley & Sons.

Beidel, D. C., Turner, S. M., & Alfano, C. (2003). Anxiety disorders. In M. Hersen, & S. M. Turner (Eds.), *Adult psychopathology and diagnosis* (4th ed.) pp. 356–419. Hoboken, NJ: John Wiley & Sons.

Block, S. D. (2000). Assessing and managing depression in the terminally ill patient. *Annals of Internal Medicine, 132*, 209–218.

Block, S. D., & Billings, J. A. (1998). Evaluating patient requests for euthanasia and assisted suicide in terminal illness: The role of the psychiatrist. In M. D. Steinberg, & S. J. Younger (Eds.), *End-of-life decisions: A psychosocial perspective* (pp. 205–233). Washington, DC: American Psychiatric Press.

Breitbart, W. (1997). The memorial delirium assessment scale. *Journal of Pain and Symptom Management, 13*(3), 128–137.

Brock, S. E. (n.d.). *Assessing psychological trauma*. Retrieved from http://www.csus.edu/indiv/b/brocks/workshops/district/ccsd.2.06.pdf

Burt, R. A. (1997). The Supreme Court speaks: Not assisted suicide but a constitutional right to palliative care. *New England Journal of Medicine, 337*, 1234–1236.

Calhoun, K. S., & Resick, P. A. (1993). Post-traumatic stress disorder. In D. H. Barlow (Ed.), *Clinical handbook of psychological disorders* (2nd ed.) (pp. 48–98). New York, NY: The Guilford Press.

Centers for Disease Control and Prevention. (2008). National hospital ambulatory medical care surbey: 2008 emergency department summary tables. Available from http://www.cdc.gov/nchs/data/ahcd/nhamcs_emergency/nhamcsed 2008.pdf

Chochinov, H. M., & Breitbart, W. (2000). *Handbook of psychiatry in palliative medicine*. New York: Oxford.

Chochinov, H., Kristejanson, L., & Hack, T. (2006). Personality, neuroticism, and coping toward the end of life. *Journal of Pain and Symptom Management, 32*(4), 332–341.

Cloninger, S. (2008). *Theories of personality: Understanding persons* (5th ed.). Upper Saddle River, NJ: Pearson/Prentice Hall.

Cook, J. M., Dinnen, S., Rehman, O., Bufka, L., & Courtois, C. (2011). Responses of a sample of practicing psychologists to questions about clinical work with trauma and interest in specialized training. *Psychological Trauma: Theory, Research, Practice, and Policy, 3*(3), 253–257.

Division of Trauma Psychology. (2010). *Division 56 Home*. Available from http://www.apatraumadivision.org/index.php

Doka, K. (1996). *Living with life threatening illness*. Washington, DC: Hospice Foundation of America.

Endicott, J. (1984, May). Measurement of depression in patients with cancer. *Cancer, 53*(10), 2243–2249.

Field, M. J., & Cassel, C. K. (Eds.). (1997). *Approaching death: Improving care at the end of life*. Washington, DC: National Academy Press.

Folstein, M., Folstein, S., & McHugh, P. (1975). Mini-mental state: A practical method for grading the cognitive state of patients for the clinician. *Journal of Psychiatric Research, 12,* 189–198.

Foti, M. E. (2003, March 9) *End-of-Life Care for Persons with Serious Mental Illness*. Powerpoint lecture presented at lecture of the Robert Wood Johnson Foundation "Do It Your Way, Promoting Excellence in End-of-Life Care," Boston, MA. Source:www.promotingexcellence.org/mentalillness.

Francis, J., Strong, S., Martin, D., & Kapoor, W. (1988). Delirium in elderly general medical patients: Common but often unrecognized [Abstract]. *Journal of Clinical Research, 36,* 711A.

Gum, A. M., King-Kallimanis, B., & Kohn, R. (2009, September). Prevalence of mood, anxiety, and substance-abuse disorders for older Americans in the national comorbidity survey-replication. *American Journal of Geriatric Psychiatry, 17*(9), 769–781.

Hayduk, L., Olson, K., Quan, H., Cree, M., & Cui, Y. (2010). Temporal changes in the causal foundations of palliative care symptoms. *Quality of Life Research, 19,* 299–306.

Herbert, R. S., Schulz, R., Copeland, V. C., & Arnold, R. M. (2009). Preparing family caregivers for death and bereavement. Insights from caregivers of terminally ill patients. *Journal of Pain and Symptom Management, 37*(1), 3–12.

International Association for the Study of Pain Task Force on Taxonomy (1994). IASP pain terminology. In H. Merskey, N. Bugduk (Eds.), *Classification of chronic pain* (2nd ed.) (pp. 209–214). Seattle, WA: IASP Press.

Jaffe, J., Segal, J., & Dumke, L. F. (2005). *Emotional and psychological trauma: Causes, symptoms, effects, and treatment*. Available from http://www.dhhs.tas.gov.au/__data/assets/pdf_file/0004/38434/Trauma.pdf

Jotkowitz, A. B., Clarfield, A. M., & Glick, S. (2005). The care of patients with dementia: A modern Jewish ethical perspective. *Journal of the American Geriatrics Society, 53*(5), 881–884.

Kessler, R. C., Chiu, W. T., Demler, O., & Walters, E. E. (2005). Prevalence, severity, and comorbidity of 12-Month DSM-IV disorders in the national comorbidity survey replication. *Archives of General Psychiatry, 62*, 617–627, doi: 10.1001/archpsyc.62.6.617.

Larson, D. G., & Tobin, D. R. (2000). End-of-life conversations: Evolving practice and theory. *Journal of American Mathematical Society, 284*(12), 1573–1578.

Lohr, I., & Cook, B. L. (2003). Mood disorders: Bipolar disorders. In M. Hersen, & S. M. Turner (Eds.), *Adult psychopathology and diagnosis* (4th ed.) (pp. 286–312). Hoboken, NJ: John Wiley & Sons.

Massachusetts Department of Mental Health. (2011). *Do it your way: Mental illness—A national problem*. Retrieved 9.19.2011 from http://www.promoting excellence.org/mentalillness/3306.html.

Maxmen, J. S., & Ward, N. G. (1995). *Essential psychopathology and its treatment*. New York: W.W. Norton and Sons.

McDade-Montez, E. A., Christensen, A. J., Cvengros, J. A., & Lawton, W. J. (2006). The role of depression symptoms in dialysis withdraw. *Health Psychology, 25*(2), 198–204.

McGuire, J. (2009). Ethical considerations when working with older adults in psychology. *Ethics & Behavior, 19*(2), 112–128.

Meeks, T. W., Vahia, I. V., Lavretsky, H., Kulkarni, G., & Jeste, D. V. (2011). A tune in "a minor" can "b major": A review of epidemiology, illness course, and public health implications of subthreshold depression in older adults. *Journal of Affective Disorders, 129*, 126–142.

Mental Health America. (2011). Depression in older adults. Retrieved September 19, 2011 from http://www.nmha.org/index.cfm?objectid=C7DF94FF-1372-4D20-C8E34FC0813A5FF9

National Institute of Mental Health. (2008a). *Any mood disorder among adults*. Retrieved September 19, 2011 from http://www.nimh.nih.gov/statistics/1ANYMOODDIS_ADULT.shtml

National Institute of Mental Health. (2008b). *Bipolar disorder among adults*. Retrieved September 19, 2011 from http://www.nimh.nih.gov/statistics/1BIPOLAR_ADULT.shtml

National Institute of Mental Health. (2008c). *Major depressive disorder among adults*. Retrieved September 19, 2011 from http://www.nimh.nih.gov/statistics/1MDD_ADULT.shtml

Newman, M. G., Szkody, L. E., Llera, S. J., & Przeworski, A. (2011). A review of technology-assisted self-help and minimal contact therapies for anxiety and depression: Is human contact necessary for therapeutic efficacy? *Clinical Psychology Review, 31*, 89–103.

Pereira, J., Hanson, J., & Bruera, E. (1997). The frequency and clinical course of cognitive impairment in patients with terminal cancer. *Cancer*, 79, 835–842.

Rainer, J. P., & Brown, F. F. (2007). *Crisis counseling and therapy*. New York: Routledge.

Rainer, J. P., & McMurry, P. E. (2002). Caregiving at the end of life. *Journal of Clinical Psychology: In Session*, 58(11), 1421–1431.

Rando, T. (1993). *Grief, dying, and death: Clinical interventions for caregivers*. Lexington, MA: Lexington Books.

U. S. Census Bureau. (2009). *2005–2009 American Community Survey 5-Year Estimates*. Retrieved October 2, 2011, from http://factfinder.census.gov/servlet/ACSSAFFFacts?_event=&geo_id=01000US&_geoContext=01000US&_street=&_county=&_cityTown=&_state=&_zip=&_lang=en&_sse=on&ActiveGeoDiv=&_useEV=&pctxt=fph&pgsl=010&_submenuId=factsheet_1&ds_name=DEC_2000_SAFF&_ci_nbr=null&qr_name=null&reg=&_keyword=&_industry=

Werth, J. L., Jr., Gordon, J. R., & Johnson, R. R., Jr. (2002). Psychosocial issues near the end of life. *Aging and Mental Health*, 6(4), 402–412.

World Health Organization (1990). *Cancer pain and palliative care: Report of a WHO expert committee. (Technical Report Series No. 804)*. Geneva, Switzerland: Author.

Young, J. E., Beck, A. T., & Weinberger, A. (1993). Depression. In D. H. Barlow (Ed.), *Clinical handbook of psychological disorders* (2nd ed.) (pp. 240–277). New York, NY: The Guilford Press.

8

Cognitive Impairment Near the End of Life

MARY M. LEWIS AND JESSICA M. MOELLER

One complicating factor for individuals who are facing the end of life is cognitive impairment, because it can influence many aspects of the end-of-life process (Richmond, Lewis, & Werth, 2010). There are no statistics that reveal the number of dying individuals across the lifespan who have or develop cognitive impairment. However, two causes of dementia, Alzheimer's disease and Parkinson's disease, were cited as the sixth and 14th leading causes of death in the United States in 2009 (Kochanek, Xu, Murphy, Minino, & Kung, 2011). It is likely that dementia and other types of cognitive impairment are even more common in dying individuals, because death certificates frequently underreport dementia as a contributing factor to death (Ganguli & Rodriguez, 1999; Sachs, Shega, & Cox-Hayley, 2004). In the United States, approximately 13.9% of adults aged 71 and over have some form of dementia (Plassman et al., 2007). Even more individuals may have temporary forms of cognitive impairment, such as delirium, that are present near the end of life but not documented as the primary cause of death.

Differentiating among various causes of impairment is important because treatment can ameliorate some conditions. For example, depression can cause an individual to have difficulty concentrating, therefore appearing to have short-term memory impairment to an observer. Successful treatment of the depression will resolve the concentration dysfunction, and therefore restore the individual to his or her baseline level of cognition. However, differential diagnosis (e.g., dementia vs. pseudodementia) is not always clear-cut as there is frequent comorbidity of conditions, especially among older adults (Patterson, 1986).

This chapter identifies the common types of cognitive impairment, as well as some general guidelines regarding differential diagnosis, and presents several cases to elucidate the importance of understanding the cognitive and emotional state of the dying individual. Cultural, legal, advocacy and policy issues are reviewed in the context of specific end-of-life concerns for the individual with cognitive impairment.

TYPES OF COGNITIVE IMPAIRMENT

Cognitive impairment can be divided into two categories: reversible (also referred to as pseudodementia) and irreversible (Patterson, 1986). Reversible cognitive impairment includes delirium, amnestic disorders, and dementia due to reversible medical conditions. Irreversible cognitive impairment tends to occur as a result of physiological damage in the brain, such as through Alzheimer's disease or stroke. Both impact the end-of-life process, but in different ways.

Reversible Cognitive Impairment

Reversible, or treatable, cognitive impairment tends to have a medical or emotional cause, and can be easily misdiagnosed if a comprehensive history and extensive medical and psychological evaluation is not conducted. If not diagnosed and treated in time, reversible cognitive impairment may result in permanent impairment. If indeed diagnosed and treated correctly, the individual may be cognitively intact enough to make competent end-of-life decisions (Richmond et al., 2010).

In the *DSM-IV-TR* (American Psychiatric Association [APA], 2000), diagnosis of reversible cognitive impairment can be categorized as delirium, dementia due to medical factors, amnestic, and other cognitive disorders (see Table 8.1). Contributing factors include acute medical issues, reactions to or interactions between medications, metabolic and endocrine disorders, acute injury, infection, substance abuse, and psychological diagnoses. Research has also found that male sex, impaired vision, and prior stroke were also risk factors (Edlund et al., 2006). Because of the possible variation, it is difficult to give a common set of symptoms. However, the typical course of a reversible cause of cognitive impairment has a rapid onset. Individuals can demonstrate disturbances in consciousness, cognition, or perception that fluctuates during the course of the illness (APA, 2000; Korevaar, van Munster, & de Rooij, 2005).

As a result of the rapid-onset of reversible cognitive impairment, individuals typically do not have advanced warning or time to discuss end-of-life options with caregivers. Unless an advanced directive already exists, an individual with reversible cognitive impairment may not be able to verbalize his or her needs directly. Unfortunately, some reversible cognitive impairment such as delirium carries with it a high risk of mortality (Edlund et al., 2006).

TABLE 8.1
Causes of Reversible Cognitive Impairment and Examples of Each

Cause	Examples
Acute medical issues	Dehydration, normal pressure hydrocephalus, malnutrition, low oxygen levels
Endocrine disorders	Hypothyroidism
Infection	Urinary tract infection (UTI), pneumonia
Injury	Concussion
Metabolic	B12 deficiency
Medication interaction	Sleep aids taken with antianxiety medication
Medication reaction	Narcotics, anesthetic
Psychological	Depression, anxiety
Substance abuse	Acute alcohol intoxication

CASE 1:

Marie was a 66-year-old woman who had a long-standing history of clinical depression and chronic pain. She was currently on an antidepressant medication and had been seeing a counselor in the community. She was also seeing a pain-management specialist for her chronic back pain. One day at home, Marie tripped on a rug, fell and broke her hip. She went through the surgery well, and came to a skilled nursing facility (SNF) for rehabilitation. While in the SNF, she was assessed by the counselor for issues related to her depression and loss of independence. She also had some pain management concerns, stating that nurses were "slow" to get her pain medications to her, and she thought the medications were not strong enough. Counseling was initiated to focus on these concerns and a cognitive-behavioral approach to therapy was used successfully to treat her depression. Marie participated fully in her physical and occupational therapy, and expressed hope she would return home.

One day Marie began to verbalize fearfulness toward the staff and developed some aggressive behaviors. She also began to ring her call light repeatedly, but was unable to identify her request once a staff member answered the call. She would request pain medications on the hour, and nursing staff reported to the counselor that she was "drug-seeking." The nursing staff also reported to the counselor that Marie had become "demanding," and assumptions were made that Marie likely had preexisting dementia that had been missed on admission. The counselor had identified some mild orientation deficits upon admission, mostly to date and time, but dismissed these are being deficits related to Marie's lack of a calendar and clock in her room. According to family, Marie had not previously shown any cognitive impairment. During counseling, Marie was unable to focus and perseverated on her pain and the difficulties she was having with the staff.

By this time, Marie had become more confused and irritable. She was unable to clearly communicate her needs and had periods of delusions that she was at work or taking a trip. She frequently complained of pain in the hip that had been broken. She was unable to meaningfully participate in counseling at this point, although she did make statements to her counselor that she was in pain, suffering, and wished to "have it all end." When clarified, she denied suicidal ideation or a wish to die, but wanted her suffering alleviated.

At the family and counselor's request, a urinalysis and bloodwork were conducted to evaluate for medical reasons for her confusion. The results revealed that Marie had developed a severe infection in her repaired hip, and that this was indeed causing both her significant pain and her cognitive impairment. Unfortunately, Marie declined rapidly despite surgical removal of her infected hip hardware and IV antibiotics. She was never referred to hospice because her family was concerned that this would contribute to her drug-seeking behavior, rather than potentially alleviate her pain and suffering. Unfortunately, because Marie came in as a healthy, young-older adult, she had not clarified her end-of-life wishes other than to state that she did not want CPR in case of cardiac arrest. She was now too confused to state her wishes, and her family was unsure as to what she wanted. Marie died within 2 weeks of the identification of her infection. According to medical staff at the facility, if Marie's bloodwork had been run a few weeks earlier, when she began showing signs of cognitive impairment, the outcome may have been different.

CLINICAL PEARL

A multidisciplinary team approach is useful when diagnosing reversible cognitive impairment. The counselor should gather a history of the cognitive and emotional baseline as well as changes in the same from family, work with the physician and nurses regarding medical diagnostic tests, and monitor both mood and changes in cognition.

Irreversible Cognitive Impairment

Irreversible cognitive impairment is frequently labeled as dementia. The most common cause of dementia is Alzheimer's disease, but there are a number of other conditions that can cause the permanent cognitive impairment known as dementia (see Table 8.2). According to the *DSM-IV-TR* (APA,

TABLE 8.2
Causes of Irreversible Cognitive Impairment and Associated Cognitive Symptoms

Cause of Irreversible Cognitive Impairment	Typical Symptoms
Alzheimer's disease	Memory impairment, language impairment, executive function impairment, apathy, disorientation
Vascular dementia	Symptoms vary depending upon location of the stroke, can include similar symptoms as Alzheimer's disease
Lewy body dementia	Memory impairment, difficulty with judgment, behavioral changes, visual hallucinations. Cognition can fluctuate between lucid and confused
Parkinson's disease	May develop in later stages of the disease process. Memory impairment, slowed thinking, hallucinations, difficulty initiating
Frontotemporal dementia	Changes in personality and behavior, language impairment
Creutzfeldt–Jakob disease	Memory impairment, impairment in motor coordination, behavioral changes
AIDS dementia complex	Memory impairment, changes in behavior and personality, disturbances in motor coordination
Huntington's disease	Personality changes

Table created with information from the Alzheimer's Association (2011) and APA (2000).

2000), dementia includes memory impairment as well as one or more of the following: language impairment, difficulty carrying out motor activities, inability to recognize people or objects, and executive function impairment. The cognitive deficits must impair social or occupational functioning. Depending upon the etiology of the dementia process, the onset may be gradual or abrupt and the course progressive, static, or remitting.

Although the symptoms are similar across various causes of dementia, differential diagnosis is critical because it allows some understanding of the progression of the cognitive decline as well as prognosis. For example, an individual who has a family history of Alzheimer's disease and who has been diagnosed early will be able to discuss end-of-life wishes with his or her family and work in counseling on emotional and end-of-life issues before significant cognitive impairment occurs (Lewis, 2007; Werth, Gordon, & Johnson, 2002). That individual may also be able to benefit from medication such as Aricept to slow down the progression of the disease, and therefore be able to benefit from counseling for a longer period of time. Keep in mind, however, that even within the subtypes of dementia, the prognosis and progression of the disease can vary widely and that each individual should be approached at the level of cognition that is present at the moment.

CASE 2:

Jerry was a 78-year-old Caucasian man who had suffered a series of strokes. After his first stroke, he demonstrated some short-term memory loss, but was able to function and live in the community with the help of his daughter and a home health worker. When he had his second and more debilitating stroke, he and his family made the decision to admit him to a long-term care (LTC) facility for 24-hour care. Jerry was paralyzed on the right side, and had mild language impairments, especially in word finding, and moderate short-term memory deficits as a result of his diagnosed vascular dementia. He also showed some emotional lability. Some days were better than others, cognitively and emotionally.

The referral to the counselor came when Jerry stated that he "wanted to be with his wife." Staff believed that this was a suicidal statement because his wife was dead, although Jerry denied suicidal ideation or means. The counselor assessed Jerry and determined that he was experiencing an adjustment disorder with depressed mood secondary to his admission to the LTC and continued grief over the loss of his wife the prior year. He also was frustrated at his trouble communicating his needs to the staff because of his word-finding deficits. Jerry was seen for counseling on days his cognition allowed it, with a focus on grief resolution and increasing his ability to cope with his limitations. The facility physician also started Jerry on an antidepressant to assist with his mood lability. In time, following a validation approach and cognitive-behavioral treatment, Jerry's depression alleviated. Staff noted that his short-term memory also improved somewhat after his depression lifted. His moods were more stable and he was able to express that his prior statement regarding his spouse was related to the fact that he "did not want to linger" and wished to have no life-prolonging measures. A Do Not Resuscitate/Comfort Care (DNR/CC) order was put into place at Jerry's request and family assent, and he noted that knowing the order was in his chart was a relief. A DNR/CC is a medical order put into place by a physician when a person decides he or she does not wish to have cardiopulmonary resuscitation (CPR) performed should the heart stop beating. Counseling was mutually terminated, although the counselor was able to informally stay in touch with Jerry while in the LTC facility for other reasons.

In time, Jerry had another stroke. This third and last stroke was more severe than the others, and Jerry was unable to speak or engage with his family or staff, and was unable to swallow. Because Jerry had previously discussed his end-of-life wishes with the counselor and his family, as well as completing the DNR/CC order, he was provided the palliative care that he requested at the LTC facility and not given a feeding tube, per his requests. According to his family and the nursing staff, he died peacefully in his bed at the facility with the picture of his wife at his side and his family present.

CLINICAL PEARL

Dementia and depression often coexist, but successful treatment of the depression can assist in returning some cognitive functioning to the point where the individual can participate in end-of-life decision making.

COUNSELING INTERVENTIONS APPROPRIATE FOR INDIVIDUALS WITH COGNITIVE IMPAIRMENT NEAR THE END OF LIFE

The type of counseling intervention selected when working with an individual with cognitive impairment near the end of life will depend on several factors, most notably the theoretical orientation of the counselor, the socioemotional and physical concerns of the individual, and the individual's level of cognitive impairment. In general, long-term approaches to counseling such as psychoanalytic treatments may be less helpful to individuals who are dying, whereas interventions that are focused on meaning making, validation, and an understanding of the grief process have been found to be useful (Connor, Lycan, & Schumacher, 2006; Kastenbaum, 2000). However, an individual with cognitive impairment may not have the ability to discuss abstract ideas such as meaning or grief in the same way as cognitively intact individuals. In fact, there is very little research on the role of counseling in individuals with dementia or delirium that focuses on end-of-life issues. Research that exists on the role of counseling with older adults who have cognitive impairment tends to focus on interventions effective for managing behavioral disturbances (e.g., Fisher, Harsin, & Hayden, 2000) rather than emotional disturbances.

The counseling interventions discussed in this section have not been empirically validated for use with individuals with cognitive impairment who are near the end of life. However, the authors have found clinical use of these tools to be beneficial, and offer them as possible interventions for the counselor's toolbox. In general, no matter the source of the cognitive impairment, an individual's ability to communicate effectively may be compromised. Therefore, beyond any specific intervention the counselor chooses, developing a strong therapeutic relationship and focusing attention to the subvocal and nonverbal aspects of communication are the most critical aspects of the counseling process (Duffy, 1999; Kastenbaum, 2000). If at all possible, the counseling process should start before significant declines in the ability to communicate occur (Kastenbaum, 2000).

The Life Review (Butler, 1963). The life review is a well-established technique in counseling older adults, and has been found to be a useful tool in finding a sense of self (see Butler, 1995; Kastenbaum, 2000). It may be that those individuals who are near the end of life can utilize the life review to face death by constructing a current sense of self that has meaning (Kastenbaum, 2000). The life review is useful for individuals with cognitive impairment because it taps into more remote memories, which may remain intact longer.

Validation Therapy (Feil, 1993, 1999). Validation therapy was specifically designed for adults over age 80 who have cognitive impairment (Feil, 1993, 1999). The therapy focuses on four phases of resolution, and is intended for individuals in the final stages of life. Empathy is the key to validation therapy, as is an understanding of the links between the physical, psychological, and social characteristics of the individual. Although Feil designed validation therapy for adults over 80 years of age, the techniques and interventions may also be useful for young-old and middle-old adults.

Play Therapy (Frey, 1993; Lewis & Trzinski, 2006). Play therapy was originally designed for use in children, but has been used with adults (Frey, 1993). The first pilot project of play therapy in older adults was designed by Trzinski and Higgins (2001). They found that in a group setting with older adults with cognitive impairment, play therapy was useful in exploration of feelings. A specific case of the use of a "group buddy" play therapy intervention in a group dealing with death is described by Lewis and Trzinski (2006) and illustrates potential efficacy of this therapeutic technique for older adults with cognitive impairment who are dealing with end-of-life issues.

Spaced Retrieval (SR; Brush & Camp, 1998; Camp, Bird, & Cherry, 2000; Lewis & Trzinski, 2006). SR is a technique traditionally used by speech therapists to help individuals with cognitive impairment learn new information and be able to recall it at a later time (Brush & Camp, 1998; Camp et al., 2000; Lewis, 1999). The technique relies on implicit memory, which is intact longer than explicit memory in individuals with dementia (Brush & Camp, 1998; Lewis, 1999). Much of the research on SR has focused on the recall of facts such as names of hospital staff or the time of lunch. Lewis and Trzinski described a female client who was grieving the loss of a niece but was unable to remember who had died. The SR technique was able to assist the client in recalling the name and relationship of the person who had died, and therefore the client was able to move forward in the grieving process. The technique can be used in the routine context of therapy, potentially to assist older adults with dementia in recalling information pertinent to the counseling process or their own end-of-life concerns (Lewis & Trzinski, 2006).

Problem-Focused Therapy. A recent study by Arean et al. (2010) explored the efficacy of problem solving and supportive therapy in older adults suffering from both executive dysfunction and major depression. Problem solving and supportive therapy were found to be equally effective in the initial stages of counseling (weeks 0–6) but differences were found at week 9 and 12 in that problem-solving therapy was more effective. Although both delirium and dementia were considered exclusion criteria in the Arean et al. study, executive dysfunction is one aspect of dementia and therefore this research may be applicable to individuals with mild forms of dementia. It is unclear as to whether problem-solving therapy would be effective with individuals who have cognitive impairment and are near the end of life.

CRITICAL ISSUES FOR INDIVIDUALS WITH COGNITIVE IMPAIRMENT NEAR THE END OF LIFE

There are a number of additional considerations for counselors to consider when working with individuals with cognitive impairment. These include culture, legal/ethical issues, insurance and regulatory issues, as well as advocacy issues.

Cultural Considerations

It is well known that the population in the United States is becoming increasingly culturally diverse. Thus, when working with individuals near the end of life, it is not uncommon for professionals to have patients whose culture is different from their own. There are many ways in which culture may play a role near the end of life. For example, cultural beliefs may impact decision making regarding life-sustaining treatment measures, decisions to complete advanced directives, or preferences on where and how to die. More specifically, with regard to cognitive impairment, an individual's culture may impact how symptoms of cognitive impairment are perceived, when or if an individual seeks treatment for these symptoms, and what constitutes "normal aging" (Chin, Negash, & Hamilton, 2011; Jervis & Manson, 2002; Mahoney, Cloutterbuck, Neary, & Zhan, 2005; Mok, Lai, Wong, & Wan, 2007).

Although multiple studies have attempted to examine the differences in prevalence and incidence rates of dementia across racial and ethnic groups, little consensus has been reached (Chin et al., 2011). The Alzheimer's Association (2010) estimates the prevalence of dementia in African Americans aged 65 and older to be twice the rate of Caucasians and the prevalence for Hispanics to be 1.5 times greater than Caucasians. In addition to genetic risk factors, it has been suggested that the racial disparities noted to date may also be caused by differences in education or literacy level. For example, Chin and colleagues suggested that the typical screening measures used to initially assess cognitive impairment (e.g., Mini-Mental Status Exam) have an unusually high false-positive rate for ethnic minorities, which could be attributed to differences in literacy rates. The differentiation between literacy versus education level is important because literacy takes into consideration the differences in education quality. Thus, the 8th grade education of an 85-year-old African American man raised in the South is not necessarily equivalent to the eigth grade education of an 85-year old Caucasian man raised in the North.

CLINICAL PEARL

When selecting cognitive screening tools, neuropsychological tests, or even counseling techniques/tools, it is important to consider the individual's cultural background and education and literacy levels before proceeding. Discussing the options directly with the patient or patient's family may also be beneficial.

Although it may be helpful to know which populations are at a higher risk for cognitive impairment, when counseling individuals near the end of life it may be more clinically useful to understand the differences in how cultures perceive cognitive impairment. One study found that initial changes in memory were perceived as "normal aging" across multiple ethnic groups including African Americans, Chinese, and Latinos (Mahoney et al., 2005). However, as cognitive impairment worsened, cultural differences emerged. Specifically in this study, African Americans focused on normalizing their loved one's symptoms and tolerating the behavioral and emotional changes, whereas the Chinese feared the stigma and shame associated with having a loved one with dementia (i.e., it is a contagious disease) and were hesitant to discuss their loved one's symptoms or seek help (Mahoney et al., 2005). Latinos tended to try and avoid upsetting their loved one by not discussing the changes until safety became an issue, at which point Latinos were quick to seek medical assistance (Mahoney et al., 2005). Another study focusing on American Indians and Native Alaskans found that tribes differed in their perception of confusion in the elderly (Jervis & Manson, 2002). For example, some viewed cognitive decline and the occasional associated hallucinations as the elder's ability to communicate with the next world, which could be seen as a normal part of the dying process or a sign that the elder is highly esteemed (Henderson & Traphagan, 2005; Jervis & Manson, 2002).

Clinically, these findings may help explain why some ethnic groups (e.g., African Americans) have more delayed diagnoses of dementia and receive delayed care (Chin et al., 2011). Cultural differences in access to health care and perceptions of the American health care system are also likely to play a role in the dementia and end-of-life care individuals receive.

CLINICAL PEARL

It is important to be aware of the potential cultural differences that exist when working with individuals near the end of life. However, it is also important to avoid stereotyping and assumptions about preferences and beliefs when near the end of life. When counseling culturally diverse individuals near the end of life, it is most important to treat them first and foremost as individuals and inquire specifically of their end-of-life beliefs.

Legal/Ethical Issues

Cognitive impairment in individuals near the end of life presents multiple ethical/legal issues in addition to the clinical issues already discussed. The American Academy of Neurology Ethics and Humanities Subcommittee (AANEHS, 1996) suggested that the ethical dilemmas vary based on the stage of one's cognitive impairment. Specifically, they suggest that in the early stages of dementia, issues of the capacity to make decisions and complete advanced directives are primary, whereas in the mid to late stages of dementia, issues related to appropriate level of medical treatment, decisions to restrain a patient, and caregivers become prominent (AANEHS).

As mentioned earlier, discussing end-of-life preferences and advance directives early on in one's work with terminal clients is the best practice for minimizing the legal/ethical issues that may arise if the patient becomes cognitively impaired to the point where the patient lacks the capacity to consent to his or her own medical treatment. The ability to participate in counseling will vary depending upon cognitive functioning on a given day, thus it is critical to establish consent to participate in treatment at the onset and reevaluate the benefit of therapy on an ongoing basis as cognitive impairment changes. For example, in the case of a patient with delirium, his or her capacity to participate in and benefit from counseling is low and she may be very resistant to treatment interventions when the illness is acute. However, once the delirium has resolved, it is important to re-evaluate the patient's desire for counseling and capacity to participate, as her situation has changed.

Finally, when an individual has been determined incompetent by the courts or clinically lacks the capacity to consent to treatment, the law identifies three possible courses of action (Webb, 1997). If the patient had previously completed (a) a living will or (b) designated a durable power of attorney, these wishes should be followed as closely as is feasible (Webb,

1997). If neither of these documents are in place, then the third option, a surrogacy or succession law, may prove useful. The surrogacy or succession law designates a hierarchy of possible decision makers (e.g., spouse, adult children, next closest adult relative) in the event that the individual is not competent to make his or her own decisions, has not designated a durable power of attorney, and/or the living will is not explicit enough to dictate what should occur in the given situation (Webb, 1997). An example of the latter would be if a patient specified that he or she does not want CPR and/or to be placed on a ventilator; however, the current situation involves artificial nutrition and hydration, a condition not addressed by the patient's living will. The hierarchy set forth by the surrogacy or succession law varies by state, and counselors are encouraged to become familiar with the laws of their own state.

Regulatory Issues

There are several regulatory issues related to Medicare that may be barriers to providing effective counseling to individuals with cognitive impairment near the end of life. Mental health claims are submitted through Medicare Part B, and Medicare Administrative Contractors (MACs) are responsible for processing those claims and creating the local coverage determinations (LCDs) related to mental health services (Centers for Medicare and Medicaid Services [CMS], 2011). This section will focus on general policies of Medicare, but counselors are encouraged to search the state-specific MAC webpage to identify the specific LCD related to mental health and psychotherapy. Please note that the only individuals who can provide psychotherapy independently through Medicare are psychologists who hold a doctoral degree, clinical social workers, nurse practitioners, clinical nurse specialists, physician assistants, or physicians (CMS, 2008).

The first potential barrier related to counseling individuals with cognitive impairment near the end of life is related to their level of cognitive impairment. Although MACs can create specific LCDs that specify this more clearly, in general, Medicare states that LCDs should include a statement related to the documentation of "the patient's capacity to participate in and benefit from psychotherapy" (U.S. Department of Health and Human Services [DHHS], 2001, p. 2). This can be interpreted to mean that the individual must have a level of communication that allows participation in the counseling process, as well as the short-term and long-term memory skills to retain information from session to session that would contribute to improvement in symptoms. Therefore, the individual's cognition must be assessed continually to evaluate for these two variables, and if the criteria are not met, Medicare may deny those services. The exact level of cognitive impairment that would exclude an individual from benefitting from counseling is not clear, and may depend on the type and nature of the cognitive impairment, as well as the skill level and interventions used by the counselor.

A second potential barrier relates to access to hospice care for individuals with cognitive impairment. Because delirium, or temporary cognitive impairment, is not seen as a terminal condition, the focus in this section will be on dementia. Despite dementia being listed as the sixth cause of death in the United States, very few individuals who die from dementia are actually enrolled in hospice care (Ewbank, 1999; Sachs et al., 2004). This is despite the fact that hospice is effective for individuals with dementia (Mitchell et al., 2007). Unfortunately, people with dementia who are enrolled in hospice spend less than 2 weeks in hospice care (Fried, 2005; DHHS, 2003). It appears that the three major issues related to dementia and enrollment in hospice are related to the difficulty of estimating a 6-month prognosis for an individual with dementia, difficulty recognizing dementia as a terminal condition, and accessing hospice in nursing homes (Lewis, 2007; Mitchell et al., 2007; Sachs et al., 2004).

The last barrier is related to access to mental health services when an individual is utilizing hospice care under Medicare and most other insurances. Once enrolled in hospice, mental health treatment is bundled under a global "counseling" label that includes counseling for mental health, diet, spiritual issues, and grief (Twillman & Lewis, 2011). Generally, those individuals providing counseling for an individual in hospice are social workers or clergy, although CMS indicates that any "qualified professional" would be eligible to provide those services (CMS Manual System, 2008; Twillman & Lewis, 2011). If the individual with cognitive impairment is enrolled in hospice, she may lack access to counseling services that focus on mental health issues because of this bundling issue. Psychotherapy can be billed outside this bundling if two criteria are met. First, the mental health diagnosis being treated must be unrelated to the diagnosis for which the individual is enrolled in hospice, and second that the hospice service agrees (Haley, Larson, Kasl-Godley, Neimeyer, & Kwilosz, 2003; Lewis, 2006).

In sum, the regulatory challenges are that the individual must be cognitively intact enough to participate in and benefit from counseling, be able to access proper end-of-life care through hospice if needed, and be able to continue counseling once enrolled in those services. These are difficult obstacles to overcome, and will require national policy changes.

Advocacy

Sachs et al. (2004) listed a number of variables that are barriers for end-of-life care for an individual with dementia, as well as some potential solutions (see Table 8.3). In general, for the individual with cognitive impairment near the

TABLE 8.3
Barriers to Excellent End-of-life Care for Patients With Dementia and Potential Remedies

Barrier	Potential Remedy
Dementia not seen as a terminal illness appropriate for palliative care approach	Educate health professionals and the public; publicize innovative models integrating palliative and primary care
Nature of advanced dementia and treatment decisions	Educate health professionals
Psychological and emotional challenges of withholding treatments such as antibiotics and tube feeding	Have physicians shape patient care plans in more palliative fashion, sharing greater portion of decision-making burden
Assessment and management of pain in cognitively impaired individuals	More broadly disseminate expert guidance on this topic
	Routinely utilize assessments by patient and caregiver, as well as observe patient
	Consider behavior change as a trigger for investigation and possible treatment of pain
Management of behavioral problems and psychiatric symptoms	Educate health professionals
	Refer to psychiatrists, geriatric psychiatrists, and other specialists
Challenging caregiver stress and bereavement issues	Educate health professionals
	Develop innovative bereavement programs
Economic and systemic disincentives for providing excellent end-of-life care to patients with dementia	Modify payment systems to align incentives
	Incorporate measures of end-of-life care for patients with dementia to quality improvement and quality measurement efforts

Reprinted with permission from Sachs, Shega, and Cox-Hayley (2004).

end of life, advocacy needs to focus on three levels: individual/family, multidisciplinary treatment team, and national policy. At the individual level, because individuals with cognitive impairment may not be able to speak for themselves as a result of impairments in language or memory, the counselor can work with the individual and the family to find a way to advocate for their wishes. It is critical, if at all possible, to discuss the individual's end-of-life wishes before the cognitive impairment is so significant that the individual cannot express his or her wishes and needs (Lewis, 2007). At the multidisciplinary treatment team level, the counselor can attempt to ensure that mental health and psychosocial factors are taken into consideration, rather than just focusing on the physical aspects of end of life (Werth et al., 2002). Especially in hospitals and nursing homes, where much of the end-of-life care is provided, communication among all parts of the care team is critical. Last, at the national policy level, there is a clear need to modify restrictions on access to hospice services for individuals with cognitive impairment as well as the limitations on use of counselors for mental health once the individual is enrolled in hospice. Increasing access to comprehensive emotional, spiritual, and physical support near the end of life may help with attaining a "good" death.

CLINICAL PEARL

There are numerous opportunities for advocacy when counseling individuals near the end of life at the individual, multidisciplinary team, and national policy levels. The counselor's ability to educate other health care professionals on the importance of psychosocial considerations near the end of life, as well as help facilitate the wishes of the cognitively impaired client, are critical to providing excellent end-of-life care.

CONCLUSION

The landscape of understanding cognitive impairment can be difficult to navigate, but is crucial for work with individuals who have cognitive deficits and are near the end of life. This requires careful consideration of the cultural, ethical, legal, regulatory, and advocacy issues that are present and can be challenging. However, assisting a client through the counseling process to be able to process and work through end-of-life issues is worth the challenge. Underneath the impairments that make communication or understanding difficult, there are individuals who have desires and wishes of their own. Counselors can assist those individuals in finding their voices to express themselves, as well as help others see the person beyond the illness.

REFERENCES

Alzheimer's Association. (2010). Alzheimer's disease facts and figures. *Alzheimer's & Dementia, 6,* 158–194.

Alzheimer's Association. (2011). Alzheimer's disease facts and figures. *Alzheimer's & Dementia, 7*(2), 1–68.

American Academy of Neurology Ethics and Humanities Subcommittee. (1996). Ethical issues in the management of the demented patient. *Neurology, 46,* 1180–1183.

American Psychiatric Association. (2000). *Diagnostic and statistical manual of mental disorders* (4th ed). Washington, DC: American Psychiatric Association.

Arean, P. A., Raue, P., Mackin, S., Kanellopoulus, D., McCulloch, C., & Alexopoulos, G. S. (2010). Problem-solving therapy and supportive therapy in older adults with major depression and executive dysfunction. *American Journal of Psychiatry, 167*, 1391–1398.

Brush, J. A., & Camp, C. J. (1998). *A therapy technique for improving memory: Spaced retrieval*. Beachwood, OH: Menorah Park Center for the Aging.

Butler, R. N. (1963). The life review: An interpretation of reminiscence in the aged. *Psychiatry, 26*, 65–76.

Butler, R. N. (1995). The life review. In G. Maddox (Ed.), *The encyclopedia of aging* (2nd ed., pp. 562–563). New York: Springer.

Camp, C. J., Bird, M. J., & Cherry, K. E. (2000). Retrieval strategies as a rehabilitation aid for cognitive loss in pathological aging. In R. D. Hill, L. Backman, & A. S. Stigsdotter-Neely (Eds.), *Cognitive rehabilitation in old age* (pp. 224–248). New York: Oxford University Press.

Centers for Medicare and Medicaid Services. (2008). *Medicare payments for part B mental health services*. MLN Matters, SE0816 Revised. Retrieved from http://www.cms.gov/mlnmattersarticles/downloads/SE0816.pdf

Centers for Medicare and Medicaid Services. (2011). *Local coverage determinations*. Retried from https://www.cms.gov/DeterminationProcess/04_LCDs.asp

Chin, A. L., Negash, S., & Hamilton, R. (2011). Diversity and disparity in dementia: The impact of ethnoracial differences in Alzheimer's disease. *Alzheimer's Disease, 25*(3), 187–195.

CMS Manual System. (2008). *Pub 100-2, Medicare Benefit Policy*, Chapter 9, Sections 40.1.4 and 40.2.3. Retrieved from http://www.medicare.gov

Connor, S. R., Lycan, J., & Schumacher, J. D. (2006). Involvement of psychologists in psychosocial aspects of hospice and end-of-life care. In J. L. Werth, Jr., & D. Blevins (Eds.), *Psychosocial issues near the end of life: A resource for professional care providers* (pp. 203–217). Washington, DC: American Psychological Association.

Duffy, M. (1999). Reaching the person behind the dementia: Treating comorbid affective disorders through subvocal and nonverbal strategies. In M. Duffy (Ed.), *Handbook of counseling and psychotherapy with older adults* (pp. 577–589). New York: Wiley & Sons.

Edlund, A., Lundstrom, M., Karlsson, S., Brannstrom, B., Bucht, G., & Gustafson, Y. (2006). Delirium in older patients admitted to general internal medicine. *Journal of Geriatric Psychiatry and Neurology, 19*, 83–90.

Ewbank, D. C. (1999). Deaths attributable to Alzheimer's disease in the United States. *American Journal of Public Health, 89*, 90–92.

Feil, N. (1993). *Validation breakthrough: Simple techniques for communicating with people with Alzheimer's-type dementia*. Baltimore, MD: Health Professions Press.

Feil, N. (1999). Current concepts and techniques in validation therapy. In M. Duffy (Ed.), *Handbook of counseling and psychotherapy with older adults* (pp. 590–613). New York: Wiley & Sons.

Fisher, J. E., Harsin, C. W., & Hayden, J. E. (2000). Behavioral interventions for patients with dementia. In V. Molinari (Ed.), *Professional psychology in long term care* (pp. 179–200). New York: Hatherleigh Press.

Frey, D. (1993). I brought my own toys today: Play therapy with adults. In T. Kottman, & C. Schaefer (Eds.), *Play therapy in action: A casebook for practitioners* (pp. 589–606). Northvale, NJ: Jason Aronson.

Fried, L. (2005). Alzheimer's and the (underused) Medicare hospice benefit. In K. J. Doka (Ed.), *Living with grief: Alzheimer's disease* (pp. 245–254). Washington, DC: Hospice Foundation of America.

Ganguli, M., & Rodriguez, E. G. (1999). Reporting of dementia on death certificates: A community study. *Journal of the American Geriatrics Society, 47*(7), 842–849.

Haley, W. E., Larson, D. G., Kasl-Godley, J., Neimeyer, R. A., & Kwilosz, D. M. (2003). Roles for psychologists in end-of-life care: Emerging models of practice. *Professional Psychology: Research and Practice, 34,* 626–633.

Henderson, J. N., & Traphagan, J. W. (2005). Cultural factors in dementia: Perspectives form the anthropology of aging. *Alzheimer's Disease and Associated Disorders, 19*(4), 272–274.

Jervis, L. L., & Manson, S. M. (2002). American Indians/Alaska natives and dementia. *Alzheimer's Disease and Associated Disorders, 16,* S89–S95.

Kastenbaum, R. (2000). Counseling the elderly dying patient. In V. Molinari (Ed.), *Professional psychology in long term care* (pp. 201–226). New York: Hatherleigh Press.

Kochanek, K. D., Xu, J., Murphy, S. L., Minino, A. M., & Kung, H. C. (2011). Deaths: Preliminary data for 2009. *National Vital Statistics Reports, 59*(4), 1–51.

Korevaar, J. C., van Munster, B. C., & de Rooij, S. E. (2005). Risk factors for delirium in acutely admitted elderly patients: A prospective cohort study. *BMC Geriatrics, 5*(6). See: http://www.biomedcentral.com/content/pdf/1471-2318-5-6.pdf

Lewis, M. M. (1999). Innovative interventions in dementia of the Alzheimer's type: Thinking outside the box. *The Ohio Psychologist, 45,* 16–18.

Lewis, M. M. (2006). Practice issues for psychologists working with end-of-life issues in long term care. *Psychologists in Long Term Care Newsletter, 20*(4), 2–5.

Lewis, M. M. (2007). End-of-life decisions for people with dementia: Issues in care and policy. In T. H. Lillie, & J. L. Werth, Jr. (Eds.), *End-of-life issues and persons with disabilities* (pp. 124–134). Austin, TX: PRO-ED.

Lewis, M. M., & Trzinski, A. L. (2006). Counseling older adults with dementia who are dealing with death: Innovative interventions for practitioners. *Death Studies, 30,* 777–787.

Mahoney, D. F., Cloutterbuck, J., Neary, S., & Zhan, L. (2005). African American, Chinese, and Latino family caregivers' impressions of the onset and diagnosis of dementia: Cross-cultural similarities and differences. *The Gerontologist, 45*(6), 783–792.

Mitchell, S. L., Kiely, D. K., Miller, S. C., Connor, S. R., Spence, C., & Teno, J. M. (2007). Hospice care for patients with dementia. *Journal of Pain and Symptom Management, 34,* 7–16.

Mok, E., Lai, C., Wong, F., & Wan, P. (2007). Living with early-stage dementia: The perspective of older Chinese people. *Journal of Advanced Nursing, 59*(6), 591–600.

Patterson, C. (1986). The diagnosis and differential diagnosis of dementia and the pseudo-dementia in the elderly. *Canadian Family Physician, 32,* 2607–2610.

Plassman, B. L., Langa, K. M., Fisher, G. G., Heeringa, S. G., Weir, D. R., Ofstedal, M. B. et al. (2007). Prevalence of dementia in the United States: The aging, demographics and memory study. *Neuroepidemiology, 29*(1–2), 125–132.

Richmond, J., Lewis, M. M., & Werth, J. L., Jr. (2010). End-of-life issues. In J. Cavanaugh, & C. K. Cavanaugh (Eds.), *Aging in America (Vol. I: Psychological aspects of aging)*. Westport, CT: Praeger.

Sachs, G. A., Shega, J. W., & Cox-Hayley, D. (2004). Barriers to excellent end-of-life care for patients with dementia. *Journal of General Internal Medicine, 19*, 1057–1063.

Trzinski, A., & Higgins, J. (2001). Therapeutic play activities: Building cohesion and socialization among nursing home residents. *Activities, Adaptation & Aging, 25*, 121–135.

Twillman, R., & Lewis, M. M. (2011). Shifting policy contexts: Using our voice. In S. H. Qualls, & J. Kasl-Godley (Eds.), *End of life and care and bereavement in older adults* (pp. 252–262). New York: Wiley & Sons.

U.S. Department of Health and Human Services. (2001). *Medicare part B payments for mental health services*. OEI-03-99-00130. Retrieved from http://oig.hhs.gov/oei/reports/oei-03-99-00130.pdf

U.S. Department of Health and Human Services. (2003). *Characteristics of hospice care discharges and their length of service: United States, 2000* (NCHS Series report 13, No. 154). Hyattsville, MD: Author.

Webb, M. (1997). *The good death: The new American search to reshape the end of life*. New York, NY: Bantam Books.

Werth, J. L., Jr., Gordon, J. R., & Johnson, R. R., Jr. (2002). Psychosocial issues near the end of life. *Aging and Mental Health, 6*, 402–412.

III

Assisting Loved Ones

9

Counseling the Caregivers of Clients Who Are Near the End of Life

DEBORAH P. WALDROP AND ABBIE M. KIRKENDALL

Caregivers of people who are near the end of life are intensely affected by the challenges of a terminal illness. They provide hands-on-care, manage pain and other symptoms, receive information and practical assistance from health care providers, and anticipate the needs of a person who is dying (Glajchen, 2004; Hudson, Aranda, & Kristjanson, 2004). Caregivers often function as the patient's advocate, judging the quality of health care that the patient is receiving, and monitoring professional care. They may harbor regret and guilt if they believe that the patient did not have the best possible care. Family caregivers need timely and accurate information, support, and communication that change with different stages of the illness (Glajchen, 2004). However, unmet needs have often been associated with caregiving for someone who is at life's end (Hudson et al., 2004). Caregiving for someone who is at life's end can have enduring effects on family members' physical, psychological, and spiritual well-being such that they can be considered "hidden patients" (Kristjanson & Aoun, 2004; Wein, 2000).

There is growing recognition that reciprocal suffering is experienced by patients and their families on the trajectory of a terminal illness (Witt-Sherman, 1998). The level of caregivers' needs and distress can meet and exceed those of the person who is dying. Family caregivers' well-being can be enhanced with counseling that facilitates coping, communication, and meaning making; helps families deal with unresolved issues; and prepares for adaptation to loss and bereavement (Aoun, Bird, Kristjanson, & Currow, 2010; Bainbridge, Krueger, Lohfeld, & Brazil, 2009; Hudson, Zordan, & Trauer, 2011; Kristjanson & Aoun, 2004).

Counseling the caregivers of clients who are near the end of life presents opportunities and challenges that are unique and distinct because it most often takes place in nonoffice settings that are not traditionally associated with counseling (e.g., intensive care units [ICU], homes, nursing homes, and hospice units). This chapter addresses caregiving in the context of life limiting or terminal illness, provides an overview of the experience of caregiving for a person who is dying, presents tools for assessment and intervention, and utilizes cases to illustrate the issues.

CAREGIVING AND THE CONTEXT FOR CARE NEAR THE END OF LIFE

The context of a loved one's life-limiting illness strongly influences caregivers' well-being during the dying process and in bereavement. Slow but steady changes have been occurring in where people die (Flory et al., 2004). Between 1989 and 2007, increasing numbers of people chose to remain at home rather than moving to an institutional setting near the end of life. In 2007, one-quarter of all deaths in the United States occurred at home (increasing from one-sixth in 1989). However, although the majority of older people express the wish to remain at home until the end of life, 20% die in nursing homes, and 61% die in hospitals (Bercovitz, Decker, Jones, & Remsburg, 2008). People who are dying often move between environments for care (e.g., hospital, nursing home, home setting, or hospice), and although the caregiving role may change, it does not end.

Factors that influence choices about the place where people choose to die include cultural beliefs, access to care, diagnosis and coexisting conditions, social support, race and ethnicity, and age. In 2007, people under age 65 were more likely to die at home (30%) than those 65 and over (24%). Older people were five times more likely to die in nursing homes than those under age 65 (National Center for Health & Statistics, 2011). Older persons most often die in the advanced stages of one or more chronic illnesses and have a longer time period to consider options for where they want to be at the end of life. Home death can be both the best and worst experience (Payne, 2010). Although some people who are dying deeply wish to remain at home to die, others fear how their death at home will affect loved ones. Family caregivers offer essential support for upholding a dying person's wishes for the place of death (Funk et al., 2010). As trends have shifted end-of-life care (EOLC) from the hospital to noninstitutional settings such as home, assisted living facilities (ALFs), nursing homes, and hospice residences, the roles of family caregivers have become more complex with multi-faceted responsibilities that many are not well prepared to assume. In all environments for care, attention to the needs of family caregivers is an essential component of optimal care at the end of life (Glajchen, 2004).

Counseling for caregivers of people who are dying is a core component of palliative care. Palliative care encompasses comprehensive physical, psychosocial, and spiritual care for people and their families as a unit for care.

Palliative care was defined by the World Health Organization (WHO) in 2002 as "an approach that improves the quality of life of patients and their families facing life-threatening illnesses, through the prevention and relief of suffering by means of early identification, assessment and treatment of pain and physical, psychosocial and spiritual symptoms" (p. 1).

Palliative care is a relatively new specialty that began with the hospice movement in the 1970s and has continued to develop, extending its breadth and depth in a variety of health care settings since that time. Since the field is relatively new, there is some lack of definitional clarity that is important to address. Several terms are used interchangeably. The terms "terminal," "life-limiting," "serious," and "advanced chronic" are all used to describe conditions that are expected to end in death. The Centers for Medicare and Medicaid (CMS, 2010) stipulate that a terminal illness is irreversible and will result in death within 6 months if it runs its normal course. For the purpose of this chapter, we define "nearing the end of life" as someone with a serious, life-threatening condition who is in the final stages of the illness.

Caregiving is the provision of assistance with the activities of daily living (ADL), which are bathing, dressing, toileting, eating, transferring, or the instrumental activities of daily living (IADL) that include shopping, food preparation, transportation, money management, using the telephone, and managing medications for a relative or friend. Caregivers typically are involved in medical decision making, provide assistance with ADLs, and coordinate treatment for people who are dying at home (Hauser & Kramer, 2004). Caregiving can be formal or informal. *Formal* caregivers are paid to provide care. Formal caregivers include nurses, aides, homemakers, physicians, and therapists. *Informal* caregivers are family, friends, and partners who assume primary caregiving responsibility and provide unpaid assistance with one or more ADL or instrumental activities. This chapter focuses on counseling informal caregivers.

An estimated 65.7 million people served as unpaid caregivers in 2008. Caregivers are most often family members (96%), and women (72%)—wives, daughters, and sisters. Notably, the term "caregiver" is professionally conceptualized and many who provide daily hands-on care do not self-identify as such. For most who engage in this intensely personal and intimate interaction, caregiving is synonymous with "caring for" a loved one and more often viewed as the final stage of a close and loving relationship.

EXPERIENCE OF CAREGIVING AT LIFE'S END

The dying process creates uncertainties about what will happen, how long it will take, and how to meet the person's physical, psychological, emotional, and spiritual needs (Makhija et al., 2011). Family caregivers have been found to experience increasing distress as the patient loses autonomy (Dumont et al., 2006). Some family members make the transition to a "new normal" but others struggle over that which they have no control and have trouble letting go of a loved one. The sense of new normalcy is a blend of continually changing needs and typical activities. The conflicting demands between caregiving and regular activities can cause family strain (Pickens, O'Reilly, & Sharp, 2010). Phillips and Reed (2010) found that people make meaning of the caregiving experience by: (1) focusing wholly on the person who is dying, catering to his or her preferences, (2) maintaining a sense of normalcy, (3) minimizing suffering and protecting the person's dignity, and (4) sacrificing to make life as good as possible.

Caregiving near the end of life has been described as unpredictable, intense, complex, frightening, and anguishing (Phillips & Reed, 2010). Caregiving for someone who has declining functional abilities involves the dissolution of familiar social boundaries. Providing personal hygiene such as bathing and incontinence care for another (especially an opposite gendered parent) has been described as awkward and as being "thrust into the abyss of someone else's dying" (Phillips & Reed, 2009, p. 80). Primary caregiving that takes place at home near the end of life has been found to be accompanied by intense, conflicting, negative, and difficult emotions such as fear and dread, anger and disillusionment, guilt and regret, anxiety, grief, and hopelessness (Funk et al., 2010). Understanding the range and intensity of caregivers' emotional responses is central for the development of a counseling relationship.

Studies have also documented the existence of satisfaction, thankfulness, pleasure, and inner strength that comes from caregiving for a loved one. Caregiving has also been characterized as a means for demonstrating love and generativity (Hudson et al., 2010; Oldham & Kristjanson, 2004; Stajduhar, 2003; Stajduhar & Davies, 1998). Caregiving can be profoundly moving, affirming, meaningful, and important for life closure and the completion of a relationship. Salmon and colleagues described the "transformative aspects of caregiving" that reduce burden and enhance a sense of gain (Salmon, Kwak, Acquaviva, Brandt, & Egan, 2005, p. 122). Counseling can facilitate these positive outcomes and growth through the experience.

Caregiving Challenges

Caregiving challenges can result from the interaction between family functioning, discrepancies between patient and caregiver needs, communication barriers that result in "conspiracies of silence," impaired concentration, caregivers' fear of bothering health care professionals, and the refusal of support (Hudson et al., 2004). Stressors such as the patient's changing needs and distress can increase the caregiver's emotional suffering

(Morasso et al., 2008). The relationship between stress and caregiver strain strongly suggests the importance of practical help in relieving the physical and emotional strain (Redinbaugh, Baum, Tarbell, & Arnold, 2003). Caregivers who have accepted the patient's illness are able to define illness-related problems in a more manageable way, feel capable of solving problems associated with care at life's end, and experience lower levels of strain (Redinbaugh et al., 2003). Counseling can help caregivers move toward acceptance.

Caregivers often become the proxy decision maker for someone who is at life's end (Schmid, Allen, Haley, & Decoster, 2010). The role of substituted decision makers can be stressful (Kutner, Bryant, Beaty, & Fairclough, 2006). Surrogate decision makers have described their motivation to become the health care proxy as stemming from advance care planning (ACP) conversations they had with loved ones (Goldstein, Back, & Morrison, 2008). Surrogates have been found to make their decisions based on: (1) conversations with a loved one about preferences, (2) written advance care directives, (3) shared experience (believing an "inner sense" would guide decisions because of shared–lived experiences with a loved one), (4) surrogates' own values and preferences about life, and (5) enlisting the help of others (Vig, Taylor, Starks, Hopley, & Fryer-Edwards, 2006). Informed decisions promote understanding about end-of-life wishes, and facilitate and support patients' decisions that are consistent with their values and preferences (Briss et al., 2004).

Close family connections remain the strongest bond near the end of life and a key determinant of good care for the person who is terminally ill. A good relationship between the person who is dying and his or her caregiver engenders better coping and more positive experiences (I. Dumont, Dumont, & Mongeau, 2008; Stajduhar, Martin, Barwich, & Fyles, 2008). People with serious illness and their caregivers agree that communication with each other about the patient's illness is important. However, disagreement about communication concerns are frequent in caregiver–patient pairs (Fried, Bradley, O'Leary, & Byers, 2005). The avoidance of family communication has been associated with avoidance of psychological distress, desire for mutual protection, and belief in positive thinking. Silence increases patients' loneliness and hopelessness, exacerbates caregivers' worry and anxiety, and prevents family members from accurately assessing patients' needs and physical conditions, which can undermine appropriate care (Zhang & Siminoff, 2003).

Family caregivers can be at risk for developing complications following the loss of the person they cared for; thus, it is important to identify factors that align with bereavement risk before the death. I. Dumont and colleagues (2008) identified factors that are associated with bereavement risk: (1) characteristics of the family caregiver and patient (e.g., attitude, past experiences, and feelings of competence), (2) symptoms of the illness (e.g., the types of symptoms and how they are managed), (3) the relational context (e.g., nature of communication and acceptance), (4) level of social and professional support, and (5) circumstances surrounding the death. The assessment of bereavement risk and arrangements for bereavement care is an important element of counseling caregivers for people who are dying.

Assessment Tools

Caregiving has myriad repercussions and has a broad ranging impact. Counseling can address practical needs for assistance, anticipatory grief, employment issues, time demands, health and emotional distress, and the caregiver's relationship with the person who is dying. Conducting a comprehensive assessment of the issues is important to identify the goals for counseling. A variety of tools are presented for use in multiple settings. Table 9.1 summarizes and presents access information.

- **Social work assessment tool (SWAT):** Designed for quick assessment at each visit to determine how well the caregiver is coping in 11 domains and to identify concerns for intervention (Reese et al., 2006).
- **Marwit Meuser caregiver grief inventory (MMCGI):** Designed to link between anticipatory grief, ambiguous loss, and barriers that family members face as a loved one is dying from dementia by measuring: (1) personal sacrifice burden, (2) heartfelt sadness and longing, and (3) worry and felt isolation (Marwit & Meuser, 2002, 2005).
- **Checklist of family relational abilities (CFRA):** Designed to help clinicians measure families' abilities to participate in caregiving at life's end. The checklist assesses family dynamics in four areas: (1) attachment bonds, (2) openness of communication regarding the current illness, (3) collaborative decision making regarding the current illness, and (4) overall level of family relational abilities (Wilkins, Quill, & King, 2009).
- **Caregivers' burden scale in end-of-life care (CBS-EOLC):** Designed to assess family caregivers' burden within the palliative care context. The questions are written to facilitate the caregiver ranking the frequency of feelings that are specific to providing EOLC for a loved one (S. Dumont, Fillion, Gagnon, & Bernier, 2008).
- **Patient dignity inventory:** Designed to measure five types of dignity-related distress: symptom distress, existential distress, dependency, peace of mind, and social support (Chochinov et al., 2008).
- **Bereavement risk index:** Designed to assess the risk of poor bereavement outcomes and support family members as a nursing home resident is dying (Kristjanson, Cousins, Smith, & Lewin, 2005).

TABLE 9.1
Assessment Tools for Counseling Caregivers of Clients Who Are Near the End of Life

Instrument	Description	Source
Social work assessmwent tool (SWAT)	An 11-item survey for assessing patients and caregivers separately; addresses the practical realities	Reese, D. J., et al. (2006). The Social Work Assessment Tool (SWAT). *Journal of Social Work in End-of-Life and Palliative Care, 2*(2), 65–95. Also available online at: http://www.nhpco.org/files/public/nchpp/SWAT_assessment_tool.pdf
Marwit Meuser caregiver grief inventory (MMCGI)	Two versions (1) A 50-item scale with three factors: (a) personal sacrifice burden, (b) heartfelt sadness and longing, (c) worry and felt isolation (2) Short form: a 18-item scale	Marwit, S. J., & Meuser, T. M. (2002). Development and initial validation of an inventory to assess grief in caregivers of persons with Alzheimer's disease. *Gerontologist, 42*(6), 751–765. (*The 50-item MMCGI appears in the article.*) Marwit, S. J., & Meuser, T. M. (2005). Development of a short form inventory to assess grief in caregivers of dementia patients. *Death Studies, 29*(3), 191–205. (*The 18-item version appears in the article and is also available online at:* http://www.hospicefoundation.org/uploads/assessment_sf.pdf)
Checklist of family relational abilities	11-item assessment that is designed to help clinicians gauge families' abilities to participate in palliative care. Assesses: attachment bonds, openness of communication about the current illness, collaborative decision making; and family relational abilities	Wilkins, V. M., et al. (2009). Assessing families in palliative care: A pilot study of family relational abilities. *Journal of Palliative Medicine, 12*(6), 517–519. (*The CFRA appears in the article.*)
Caregivers' burden scale in end-of-life care (CBS-EOLC)	A 16-item self-report questionnaire assessing caregiver burden	Dumont, S., Fillion, L., Gagnon, P., & Bernier, N. (2008). A new tool to assess family caregivers' burden during end-of-life care. *Journal of Palliative Care 24*(3), 151–161. (*The CBS-EOLC appears in the article.*)

(continued)

TABLE 9.1 (*continued*)

Instrument	Description	Source
Patient dignity inventory	Measures sources of dignity-related distress conceptualized as five factors: symptom distress, existential distress, dependency, peace of mind, and social support.	Chochinov, H. M., Hassard, T., McClement, S., Hack, T., Kristjanson, L. J., Harlos, M., … Murray, A. (2008). The patient dignity inventory: A novel way of measuring dignity-related distress in palliative care. *Journal of Pain and Symptom Management, 36*(6), 559–571. (The PDI appears in the article.)
Bereavement risk inventory	35-item assessment of risk in caregivers of nursing home residents who are dying	Davidson, K. M. (2003). Evidence-based protocol. Family bereavement support before and after the death of a nursing home resident. *Journal of Gerontological Nursing, 29*(1), 10–18. (The Bereavement Risk Inventory appears in the paper.)

Interventions

Structured interventions have been developed to assist caregivers for people who are near the end of life in dealing with different sources of strain. The first four interventions underscore the distinct nature of counseling that occurs when death is approaching.

- **Presence:** A counselor's compassionate acceptance of the caregiver's feelings and experience that is signaled by the willingness to remain present, which encourages the expression of intense emotions (Rando, 1984).
- **Listening to the silence:** Counselors can gather important information from caregivers' silence. The meaning of silence is illustrated in the words of a physician: "The long silence that ensued was deafening. He simply couldn't speak for minutes on end and I began to realize that his silence was telling me what (she) meant to him" (Bearden, Childers, Howell, & Palmore, 2011, p. 105).
- **Nonabandonment:** Counselors can communicate nonabandonment through specific supportive statements that honor the patient's wishes, ensure comfort, and demonstrate openness to comments about dying (West, Engelberg, Wenrich, & Curtis, 2005).
- **Psychoeducation:** Counselors can provide printed or electronic material about the illness, symptom management, or resources for caregivers

who may not be able to recall verbal information in the intensity of the situation (Hudson, Remedios, & Thomas, 2010).

Table 9.2 summarizes the following structured interventions and provides access information.

- **Advance care planning (ACP):** ACP involves conversations about end-of-life wishes. Often guided by the use of an advance directive form, these conversations are most effective when they are responsive to patient/family emotions and focus more on goals for care than on the desire for specific treatments (Tulsky, 2005). ACP can prepare a caregiver for the need to step into the role of making decisions for a loved one who is no longer able to articulate his or her choices.
- **Family–provider conferences:** Formal, structured provider-guided meetings are arranged to provide information, answer questions, and make decisions. Curtis and colleagues (2001) presented a framework for family conferences in the ICU: (1) introductions, (2) informational exchange, (3) discussions of the future, (4) decisions, (5) discussions of dying and death, and (6) closing. An alternate guiding framework includes: (1) goals for the conference, (2) who participates, and (3) how to prepare (Moneymaker, 2005).
- **The question prompt sheet (QPS):** This identifies questions that caregivers may have, to prompt discussion of important items (Hebert, Schulz, Copeland, & Arnold, 2009).
- **Family-focused grief therapy (FFGT):** FFGT is a brief, focused treatment that is designed for families who are at high risk of poor functioning during bereavement. It has four key aims: to enhance cohesiveness, communication, and conflict resolution, and to promote the expression of grief. There are five stages: (1) assessment of family functioning, (2) engagement or identifying the concerns, (3) focused treatment on problem solving, (4) consolidation or the affirmation of changed family functioning, and (5) termination (Chan, O'Neill, McKenzie, Love, & Kissane, 2004; Kissane & Bloch, 2002).
- **Dignity therapy (DT):** DT is a therapeutic life history interview that is designed to address psychosocial distress in people who are terminally ill. It is a brief, individualized approach that invites patients to talk about what is most important to them and how they want to be remembered. The discussions are recorded, transcribed, and edited into a generativity document that is given to the family. DT is a therapeutic intervention that lessens suffering and distress for caregivers of people who are terminally ill (Chochinov et al., 2005, 2011; McClement et al., 2007).
- **Living with hope program (LWHP):** LWHP is a brief intervention that is guided by a hope video and activity entitled "Stories of the Present" that is designed to foster hope in caregivers of family members (Duggleby et al., 2007).

TABLE 9.2
Interventions for Counseling Caregivers of a Client Who Is Near Death

Intervention	Dynamic	Source
Family–provider conferences	Guidelines for conducting formal family–provider communication, giving information and making decisions	Moneymaker, K. (2005). The family conference. *Journal of Palliative Medicine 8*(1), 157. (*Guidelines appear in the article.*) Curtis, J. R. (2002). Studying communication about end-of-life care during the ICU family conference: Development of a Framework. *Journal of Critical Care, 17*(3), 147–160. (*The conceptual framework appears in the article.*)
The question prompt sheet (QPS)	15 questions to identify caregivers' questions; prompt discussion	Hebert, R. S., et al. (2009). Pilot testing of a question prompt sheet to encourage family caregivers of cancer patients and physicians to discuss end-of-life issues. *American Journal of Hospice & Palliative Medicine, 26*(1), 24–32. (*The QPS appears in the article.*)
Family focused grief therapy (FFGT)	A comprehensive model of family care with a step-by-step approach to assessment and intervention	Kissane, D. W., & Bloch, S. (2002). *Family focused grief therapy.* New York: Open University Press. (*The stages of the protocol are described in the book.*)
Dignity therapy (DT) protocol	Designed to address psychosocial and existential distress; important issues are recorded into a generativity document that is shared with caregivers	Chochinov, H. M. et al. (2011). Effect of dignity therapy on distress and end-of-life experience in terminally ill patients: A randomized control trial. *Lancet Oncology, 12*(8), 753–63. For more resources see dignityincare.mb.ca. (*The protocol appears in the article.*)
Living with hope program (LWHP)	Construction of a legacy (scrapbook or audiotaped stories) with caregivers	Duggleby, W., et al. (2007). Developing a living with hope program for caregivers of family members with advanced cancer. *Journal of Palliative Care, 23*(1), 24–31. (*The protocol is outlined in the article.*)
Legacy	Designed to decrease caregiving stress and increase communication	Allen, R. S., et al. (2008). Legacy activities as interventions approaching the end of life.

(continued)

9. Counseling the Caregivers of Clients Who Are Near the End of Life 195

TABLE 9.2 (*continued*)

Intervention	Dynamic	Source
		Journal of Palliative Medicine, 11(7), 1029–1038. (*The protocol is outlined in the article*.)
Reminiscence	To promote expression of the feelings of grief and facilitate the process of grieving	Rando, T. A. (1984). The family of the dying patient. *Grief, dying and death: Clinical interventions with caregivers* (pp. 327–365). Champagne, IL: Research Press Company. (*A 4-stage protocol appears in the chapter*.)

- **Legacy:** This family-based intervention is designed to decrease caregiving stress and increase family communication among individuals with chronic, life-limiting illnesses, and their family caregivers. Three home visits are used to construct a personal legacy, scrapbook with photographs, or audiotaped stories (Allen, Hilgeman, Ege, Shuster, & Burgio, 2008).
- **Reminiscence:** Reminiscence therapy aims to promote expression of all the feelings of grief and to facilitate the process of grieving. Rando (2000) presented a four-phase model for intervention with anticipatory mourning: (1) assessment of the family network, the illness, and approaching death, (2) triage how the course of the illness affects the person, (3) treatment focused on the seven generic operations of anticipatory mourning, and (4) follow-up after the death.

CASE 1: DEPENDENCE AND GUILT AT LIFE'S END

Donald (age 85) and Mary Ann (age 83) Thomas have been married for 65 years. Donald suffered a stroke and entered the nursing facility 3 months later after falling at home and fracturing his right hip.

Mr. Thomas could not walk without assistance or dress himself. He had difficulty feeding himself and suffered from poor vision. The stroke left him extremely weak, and he was confined to a wheelchair. He continued to recognize his family, but became increasingly confused to place and time. With recognition that Mr. Thomas was demonstrating physical and functional decline, the nursing home staff made a referral to hospice. The social worker in this case was employed by the hospice.

Mary Ann and Donald had one daughter Susan, who lived across the country, was married and had two children, ages 2 and 4. Susan was a stay-at-home mom whose husband had recently lost his job. Susan and her family were financially unable to travel to assist Mary Ann and

Donald. Susan spoke with her mother once a day and provided emotional support over the phone. She felt a tremendous guilt for not being able to be physically present to assist with caregiving duties. She discussed her intense guilt with the hospice social worker.

Mary Ann was diagnosed with multiple sclerosis at age 32 and needed to use a wheelchair at age 58. Donald and Mary Ann had done everything together. Mary Ann never worked outside the home. Mary Ann was unable to care for Donald's complex medical needs because of her own frailty and, as a result, she had to arrange for Donald to remain in the nursing home. Mary Ann felt extremely guilty that she was not able to care for Donald at home. She thought that if the roles were reversed, Donald would have provided enough care so that she would not have had to be in a nursing home. Mary Ann was also overwhelmed by taking care of the house. She had never balanced her bank account before or paid bills and she was unable to drive. A next door neighbor had been driving her to see her husband and to take her to appointments. Mary Ann also felt resentment because she had thought she would die before Donald and she had wanted him to be there to take care of her. She began to fear her future. She shared these feelings with the hospice social worker.

Counseling Issues

Mary Ann's feelings of intense guilt about not being able to care for her husband the way he cared for her became a barrier to dealing with her anticipatory loss and needs as Donald approaches life's end. Mary Ann's resentment of Donald's decline became a barrier for addressing her own decision making about the end of life. Mary Ann also felt overwhelmed with taking care of the house.

Action Taken

The social worker worked with Mary Ann to understand that caring for her husband encompassed far more than his physical needs. Another aspect of counseling was to help her acknowledge that the physical challenges that prevented her from caring for her husband were out of her control. However, she could still be present with him and be there for emotional support. The social worker and Mary Ann listed all the ways she could support her husband emotionally, building on their 65 years of marriage and shared history.

The social worker addressed Mary Ann's resentment by validating her anger about the current situation and then empowered Mary Ann by having her recall circumstances in which she independently addressed an issue or concern. The social worker encouraged her to maintain her friendships and to make lunch dates and provided contact information for senior transport services. Mary Ann and Donald had the financial means for hiring a lawn service. The space social worker introduced the idea of moving into an assisted living facility so that Mary Ann could decrease her household responsibilities, receive the additional support she needed, and have more opportunity to socialize.

Outcome

Although Mary Ann had always been dependent on Donald, she was able to tell the social worker that she and her husband did not have a strong emotional connection. She described her husband as the *"strong, silent type."* It was difficult for her to conceive of how to support her husband emotionally. The social worker struggled with helping Mary Ann to develop her independence. Mary Ann was very fearful of taking public transportation on her own and did not have many friends.

Susan

Susan struggled with her husband's unemployment and her guilt about not being able to provide direct support to her parents. The social worker had a weekly telephone counseling session with Susan. During these calls, Susan received updates on her father's condition. The social worker also organized conference calls for family meetings with the hospice team. Susan called her father daily. Periodically, the social worker utilized a laptop for Donald so that he was able to see his grandchildren over Skype.

Despite the suggestions made, Susan struggled with guilt about not being able to afford to travel to help her mother. The social worker would regularly talk with Susan about her guilt, brainstorming ways she could provide support from a distance.

CASE 2: ADDICTION AND ESTRANGEMENT AT LIFE'S END

Gerald (Gerry) Smith was a 70-year-old who had had Parkinson's disease since he was 44 years old. He had a stroke at age 60. Gerry was in a wheelchair and the Parkinson's disease had advanced to the point that his ability to swallow had become severely limited. The combination of his medications and alcoholism took a toll on his liver. He became jaundiced and demonstrated mild confusion, which are signs of liver failure. Gerry's physician made a referral to hospice.

Gerry had been divorced since he was 32 years old and never remarried. He had one son, Bret who is 40 years old, single, and lives 6 hours away. Bret and Gerry were estranged. Bret had regular contact with the hospice social worker to get updates on his father's condition but refused to be his father's health care proxy or his power of attorney. Bret explained that he just could not be part of his father's life because he was tired of the lies and manipulation. The social worker focused with Gerry on identifying the positive outcomes of having contact with Bret before Gerry died. The social worker emphasized that Bret was Gerry's legacy and asked how Gerry wanted Bret to remember him.

Bret exhibited a high level of self-awareness and explained that he knew that his lack of a relationship with his father had affected every relationship in his life. He had tried to reconcile with his father on several occasions but inevitably Gerry would lie or manipulate the situation to get money. Bret shared that it was tiring to constantly police what his father's motives were. He thought that cutting ties with his father was less distressing than having him in his life. Bret talked about how he would feel if his father passed without having had the chance for closure.

Action Taken

The social worker utilized Bret's self-awareness and asked Bret to reflect on how his father's death without closure would impact his future relationships. The social worker utilized role plays with Bret and allowed him to verbalize what he would like to say to his father. The social worker encouraged Bret to write a letter to his father and to express his thoughts and feelings on paper.

Outcome

Bret met with his father. The social worker counseled Bret on how to approach this final conversation. She worked with Bret to maintain his boundaries and to protect himself while also being able to forgive his father. She worked with Gerry on how to apologize to his son and to tell him that he loved him. The conversation was difficult but represented some amount of closure for both. Bret was at risk for complicated grief and the social worker explained the benefits of working with a grief counselor to address and work through some of his unresolved feelings in bereavement.

CONCLUSION

Counseling caregivers of people who are nearing the end of life is an essential component of quality care and a fundamental element of palliative care. Family members who move into the role of providing hands-on assistance with increasing numbers of ADLs as well as emotional support, and who ultimately become decision makers for a loved one, can experience intense emotions and distress. Counseling is important to help caregivers cope with the often intensifying challenges, insecurity, and anxiety that accompany a loved one's decline. Although counseling is important to help caregivers during the dying process, it can also have long-term benefits in preparing family members for bereavement and life after the person's death.

The importance of a thorough and accurate assessment before beginning counseling with caregivers cannot be overstated. Effective counseling is facilitated by an assessment of individual and family dynamics, the social and medical context, and accurate knowledge of the dying person's illness trajectory and prognosis. Assessment may take different forms depending on the environment for care (e.g., home, hospital, nursing home, or hospice). In addition, assessment needs to differ by type of illness. Since time is often of the essence when working with people who are nearing death and their caregivers, formal assessment tools can expedite the process. The assessment tools in Table 9.1 are an important starting point for the field, yet additional situation-specific tools are needed. Moreover, development of sensitive assessment tools that are culturally relevant is important.

Counselors who work with people who are nearing death and their caregivers have the privilege and opportunity for helping families complete their work and prepare for the final stage of their relationships. Being present and listening are simple yet paramount to effective interventions. Counselors may work with caregivers alone, helping to decrease distress and enhance coping. However, counselors may also work with the caregiver and person who is dying to resolve psychosocial and existential distress and to facilitate the process of grieving. The interventions presented in Table 9.2 offer some specific ideas; additional evidence-based interventions for differential situations are needed. Communication is a common theme; clearly assisting and facilitating open communication about the complex and difficult issues that families often struggle to put into words can help people grieve and work toward resolution. Counseling the caregivers of people who are near the end of life is a tremendously meaningful work that can have a powerful effect on caregivers' well-being and mental health for the rest of their lives.

REFERENCES

Allen, R. S., Hilgeman, M. M., Ege, M. A., Shuster, J. L., Jr., & Burgio, L. D. (2008). Legacy activities as interventions approaching the end of life. *Journal of Palliative Medicine, 11*(7), 1029–1038.

Aoun, S., Bird, S., Kristjanson, L. J., & Currow, D. (2010). Reliability testing of the FAMCARE-2 scale: Measuring family carer satisfaction with palliative care. *Palliative Medicine, 24*(7), 674–681.

Bainbridge, D., Krueger, P., Lohfeld, L., & Brazil, K. (2009). Stress processes in caring for an end-of-life family member: Application of a theoretical model. *Aging & Mental Health, 13*(4), 537–545.

Bearden, D. M., Childers, T., Howell, S., & Palmore, J. (2011). Lessons from the silence. *Journal of Palliative Medicine, 14*(1), 105–106.

Bercovitz, A., Decker, F. H., Jones, A. L., & Remsburg, R. (2008). End-of-life care in nursing homes: 2004 National Nursing Home Survey. *National Health Statistics Report, 9*, 2–24.

Briss, P., Rimer, B., Reilley, B., Coates, R. C., Lee, N. C., Mullen, P. et al. (2004). Promoting informed decisions about cancer screening in communities and healthcare systems. *American Journal of Preventive Medicine, 26*(1), 67–80.

Centers for Medicare and Medicaid Services. (2010). *Medicare hospice utilization by state calendar year 2009*. Retrieved from https://www.cms.gov/DataCompendium/15_2009_Data_Compendium.asp

Chan, E. K. H., O'Neill, I., McKenzie, M., Love, A., & Kissane, D. W. (2004). What works for therapists conducting family meetings: Treatment integrity in family-focused grief therapy during palliative care and bereavement. *Journal of Pain & Symptom Management, 27*(6), 502–512.

Chochinov, H. M., Hack, T., Hassard, T., Kristjanson, L. J., McClement, S., & Harlos, M. (2005). Dignity therapy: A novel psychotherapeutic intervention for patients near the end of life. *Journal of Clinical Oncology, 23*(24), 5520–5525.

Chochinov, H. M., Hassard, T., McClement, S., Hack, T., Kristjanson, L. J., Harlos, M., & Murray, A. (2008). The patient dignity inventory: A novel way of measuring dignity-related distress in palliative care. *Journal of Pain & Symptom Management, 36*(6), 559–571.

Chochinov, H. M., Kristjanson, L. J., Breitbart, W., McClement, S., Hack, T. F., Hassard, T. et al. (2011). Effect of dignity therapy on distress and end-of-life experience in terminally ill patients: A randomised controlled trial. *Lancet Oncology, 12*(8), 753–762.

Curtis, J. R., Patrick, D. L., Shannon, S. E., Treece, P. D., Engelberg, R. A., & Rubenfeld, G. D. (2001). The family conference as a focus to improve communication about end-of-life care in the intensive care unit: Opportunities for improvement. *Critical Care Medicine, 29*(2 Suppl), N26–N33.

Duggleby, W., Wright, K., Williams, A., Degner, L., Cammer, A., & Holtslander, L. (2007). Developing a living with hope program for caregivers of family members with advanced cancer. *Journal of Palliative Care, 23*(1), 24–31.

Dumont, I., Dumont, S., & Mongeau, S. (2008). End-of-life care and the grieving process: Family caregivers who have experienced the loss of a terminal-phase cancer patient. *Qualitative Health Research, 18*(8), 1049–1061.

Dumont, S., Fillion, L., Gagnon, P., & Bernier, N. (2008). A new tool to assess family caregivers' burden during end-of-life care. *Journal of Palliative Care, 24*(3), 151–161.

Dumont, S., Turgeon, J., Allard, P., Gagnon, P., Charbonneau, C., & Vezina, L. (2006). Caring for a loved one with advanced cancer: Determinants of psychological distress in family caregivers. *Journal of Palliative Medicine, 9*(4), 912–921.

Flory, J., Yinong, Y.-X., Gurol, I., Levinsky, N., Ash, A., & Emanuel, E. (2004). Place of death: U.S. trends since 1980. *Health Affairs, 23*(3), 194–200.

Fried, T. R., Bradley, E. H., O'Leary, J. R., & Byers, A. L. (2005). Unmet desire for caregiver–patient communication and increased caregiver burden. *Journal of the American Geriatrics Society, 53*(1), 59–65.

Funk, L. M., Stajduhar, K. I., Toye, C., Aoun, S., Grande, G., & Todd, C. (2010). Part 2: Home-based family caregiving at the end of life: A comprehensive review of published qualitative research (1998–2008). *Palliative Medicine, 24*(6), 594–607.

Glajchen, M. (2004). The emerging role and needs of family caregivers in cancer care. *The Journal of Supportive Oncology, 2*(2), 145–155.

Goldstein, N. E., Back, A. L., & Morrison, R. S. (2008). Titrating guidance: A model to guide physicians in assisting patients and family members who are facing complex decisions. *Archives of Internal Medicine, 168*(16), 1733–1739.

Hauser, J. M., & Kramer, B. J. (2004). Family caregivers in palliative care. *Clinics in Geriatric Medicine, 20*(4), 671–688.

Hebert, R. S., Schulz, R., Copeland, V. C., & Arnold, R. M. (2009). Pilot testing of a question prompt sheet to encourage family caregivers of cancer patients and physicians to discuss end-of-life issues. *American Journal of Hospice & Palliative Medicine, 26*(1), 24–32.

Hudson, P. L., Aranda, S., & Kristjanson, L. J. (2004). Meeting the supportive needs of family caregivers in palliative care: Challenges for health professionals. *Journal of Palliative Medicine, 7*(1), 19–25.

Hudson, P. L., Remedios, C., & Thomas, K. (2010). A systematic review of psychosocial interventions for family carers of palliative care patients. *BMC Palliative Care, 9*(17), 1–6.

Hudson, P. L., Trauer, T., Graham, S., Grande, G., Ewing, G., Payne, S. et al. (2010). A systematic review of instruments related to family caregivers of palliative care patients. *Palliative Medicine, 24*(7), 656–668.

Hudson, P. L., Zordan, R., & Trauer, T. (2011). Research priorities associated with family caregivers in palliative care: International perspectives. *Journal of Palliative Medicine, 14*(4), 397–401.

Kissane, D. W., & Bloch, S. (Eds.). (2002). *Family focused grief therapy*. New York: Open University Press.

Kristjanson, L. J., & Aoun, S. (2004). Palliative care for families: Remembering the hidden patients. *Canadian Journal of Psychiatry—Revue Canadienne de Psychiatrie, 49*(6), 359–365.

Kristjanson, L. J., Cousins, K., Smith, J., & Lewin, G. (2005). Evaluation of the bereavement risk index (BRI): A community hospice care protocol. *International Journal of Palliative Nursing, 11*(12), 610.

Kutner, J. S., Bryant, L. L., Beaty, B. L., & Fairclough, D. L. (2006). Symptom distress and quality-of-life assessment at the end of life: The role of proxy response. *Journal of Pain & Symptom Management, 32*(4), 300–310.

Makhija, S. K., Gilbert, G. H., Clay, O. J., Matthews, J. C., Sawyer, P., & Allman, R. M. (2011). Oral health-related quality of life and life-space mobility in community-dwelling older adults. *Journal of the American Geriatrics Society, 59*(3), 512–518.

Marwit, S. J., & Meuser, T. M. (2002). Development and initial validation of an inventory to assess grief in caregivers of persons with Alzheimer's disease. *Gerontologist, 42*(6), 751–765.

Marwit, S. J., & Meuser, T. M. (2005). Development of a short form inventory to assess grief in caregivers of dementia patients. *Death Studies, 29*(3), 191–205.

McClement, S., Chochinov, H. M., Hack, T., Hassard, T., Kristjanson, L. J., & Harlos, M. (2007). Dignity therapy: Family member perspectives. *Journal of Palliative Medicine, 10*(5), 1076–1082.

Moneymaker, K. (2005). The family conference. *Journal of Palliative Medicine, 8*(1), 157.

Morasso, G., Costantini, M., Di Leo, S., Roma, S., Miccinesi, G., Merlo, D. F. et al. (2008). End-of-life care in Italy: Personal experience of family caregivers. A content analysis of open questions from the Italian Survey of the Dying of Cancer (ISDOC). *Psycho-Oncology, 17*(11), 1073–1080.

National Center for Health Statistics. (2011). *Health, United States 2010: With special features on death and dying* (p. 63). Hyattsville, MD: Author. Available at http://www.cdc.gov/nchs/data/hus/hus10.pdf

Oldham, L., & Kristjanson, L. J. (2004). Development of a pain management programme for family carers of advanced cancer patients. *International Journal of Palliative Nursing, 10*(2), 91–99.

Payne, S. (2010). White Paper on improving support for family carers in palliative care: Part 1. *European Journal of Palliative Care, 15*(5), 238–245.

Phillips, L. R., & Reed, P. G. (2009). Into the Abyss of someone else's dying: The voice of the end-of-life caregiver. *Clinical Nursing Research, 18*(1), 80–97.

Phillips, L. R., & Reed, P. G. (2010). End-of-life caregiver's perspectives on their role: Generative caregiving. *Gerontologist, 50*(2), 204–214.

Pickens, N. D., O'Reilly, K. R., & Sharp, K. C. (2010). Holding on to normalcy and overshadowed needs: Family caregiving at end of life. *Canadian Journal of Occupational Therapy—Revue Canadienne d Ergotherapie, 77*(4), 234–240.

Rando, T. A. (1984). *Grief, dying and death: Clinical interventions for caregivers* (pp. 75–117). Champaign, IL: Research Press Company.

Rando, T. A. (2000). Promoting healthy anticipatory mourning in intimates of the life-threatened or dying person. In Rando, T. A. (Ed.), *Clinical dimensions of anticipatory mourning* (pp. 307–378). Champaign, IL: Research Press.

Redinbaugh, E. M., Baum, A., Tarbell, S., & Arnold, R. (2003). End-of-life caregiving: What helps family caregivers cope? *Journal of Palliative Medicine, 6*(6), 901–909.

Reese, D. J., Raymer, M., Orloff, S. F., Gerbino, S., Valade, R., Dawson, S. et al. (2006). The social work assessment tool (SWAT). *Journal of Social Work in End-of-Life and Palliative Care, 2*(2), 65–95.

Salmon, J. R., Kwak, J., Acquaviva, K. D., Brandt, K., & Egan, K. A. (2005). Transformative aspects of caregiving at life's end. *Journal of Pain and Symptom Management, 29*(2), 121–129.

Schmid, B., Allen, R. S., Haley, P. P., & Decoster, J. (2010). Family matters: Dyadic agreement in end-of-life medical decision making. *Gerontologist, 50*(2), 226–237.

Stajduhar, K. I. (2003). Examining the perspectives of family members involved in the delivery of palliative care at home. *Journal of Palliative Care, 19*(1), 27–35.

Stajduhar, K. I., & Davies, B. (1998). Palliative care at home: Reflections on HIV/AIDS family caregiving experiences. *Journal of Palliative Care, 14*(2), 14–22.

Stajduhar, K. I., Martin, W. L., Barwich, D., & Fyles, G. (2008). Factors influencing family caregivers' ability to cope with providing end-of-life cancer care at home. *Cancer Nursing, 31*(1), 77–85.

Tulsky, J. A. (2005). Beyond advance directives: Importance of communication skills at the end of life. *Journal of the American Medical Association, 294*(3), 359–365.

Vig, E. K., Taylor, J. S., Starks, H., Hopley, E. K., & Fryer-Edwards, K. (2006). Beyond substituted judgment: How surrogates navigate end-of-life decision-making. *Journal of the American Geriatrics Society, 54*(11), 1688–1693.

Wein, S. (Ed.). (2000). *The family in terminal illness* (2nd ed.). New York: John Wiley & Sons, Ltd.

West, H. F., Engelberg, R. A., Wenrich, M. D., & Curtis, J. R. (2005). Expressions of nonabandonment during the intensive care unit family conference. *Journal of Palliative Medicine, 8*(4), 797–807.

WHO. (2002). *Definition of palliative care*. Retrieved May 5, 2011, from http://www.who.int/cancer/palliative/definition/en/

Wilkins, V. M., Quill, T. E., & King, D. A. (2009). Assessing families in palliative care: A pilot study of the checklist of family relational abilities. *Journal of Palliative Medicine, 12*(6), 517–519.

Witt-Sherman, D. (1998). Reciprocal suffering: The need to improve caregivers' quality of life through palliative care. *Journal of Palliative Medicine, 1*(4), 357–366.

Zhang, A. Y., & Siminoff, L. A. (2003). Silence and cancer: Why do families and patients fail to communicate? *Health Communication, 15*(4), 415–429.

10

Complicated Grief and the End of Life: Risk Factors and Treatment Considerations

ROBERT A. NEIMEYER AND LAURIE A. BURKE

CASE 1:

Some 18 months after the death of her husband, Mary, age 62, describes herself as "drowning in a sea of grief." Far from moving toward some form of recovery, she experiences herself as "stuck" in a futile protest against the impossibility of living without John, who had been the "compass" for her life for the past two decades. Without the special caring, attunement, and structure he provided her, Mary feels "disoriented," "unreal," as if his death is "just some sort of terrible joke" on the part of a cruel or neglectful God. John's relatively fast demise from an aggressive cancer gave her little time to adapt to the harsh reality of his impending loss, but Mary confesses that she spent the majority of this "warning period" actively resisting the knowledge of his eventual death and "struggling" with other family members regarding whether to continue aggressive treatment in the face of "unrealistic hope" offered by his doctors. Now, she feels deeply lonely and "cut off" from others, with the exception of her concerned adult daughter, and is caught up in an angry dispute with John's children by another marriage about the estate. Tearfully, she describes how she has "no purpose for living" since his death, and although she is not actively suicidal, she finds herself wishing that it were she, rather than he, who had died.

Few people go through life without experiencing grief as a result of the loss of a loved one, with each death leaving on average six or more significant others in its wake (McDaid, Trowman, Golder, Hawton, & Sowden, 2008). Bereavement, however, is variable in both its course and its consequences. In terms of duration, significant grief may be limited to a few weeks in the case of individuals who are highly resilient (Bonanno

& Kaltman, 2001), though a more normative trajectory involves readjustment to life over the course of a few years (Bonanno, Wortman, & Nesse, 2004). On the extreme end of the continuum, *complicated grief* (CG; Prigerson et al., 1995; Shear et al., 2011) or *prolonged grief disorder* (PGD; Boelen & Prigerson, 2007)—a reaction to loss that is marked by protracted, debilitating, sometimes life-threatening symptomatology (Latham & Prigerson, 2004)—affects approximately 10% to 15% of the population who are not bereaved as a result of violence (Prigerson et al., 1995), though a far higher incidence of complication characterizes those bereaved because of violence (McDevitt-Murphy, Neimeyer, Burke, & Williams, 2012; Shear, Jackson, Essock, Donahue, & Felton, 2006), as well as those who lose children (Keesee, Currier, & Neimeyer, 2008). Our goal in this chapter is to draw attention to features of CG that should concern clinicians working with families grieving the death of a loved one, and to underscore empirically supported risk factors for this extended and debilitating condition. We will also note recent work that attempts to bridge challenges encountered in the course of end-of-life (EOL) care with those evident in bereavement among surviving family members. Finally, we will discuss some interventions in the course of palliative and hospice care that hold promise for mitigating suffering of family members following their loved one's death, and will close by noting some principles and practices that can inform grief therapy for those whose grief is extended and life damaging.

FEATURES OF COMPLICATED GRIEF

As exemplified in Mary's case, CG is characterized by a relentless period of profound grieving that continues for at least 6 months beyond the death of the loved one, in which the survivor suffers marked and disruptive separation distress and psychologically disturbing and intrusive thoughts of the deceased. Additionally, CG frequently entails a sense of emptiness and meaninglessness about life and/or the future, trouble accepting the reality of the loss, and difficulty moving forward in making a life without the deceased (Holland, Neimeyer, Boelen, & Prigerson, 2009; Prigerson & Jacobs, 2001). Stroebe, Schut, and Stroebe (2007) found that grievers, especially spouses, have an increased risk of early mortality merely as a result of being bereaved, and other investigators have found CG in particular to predict a variety of concerning conditions, including impaired quality of life and social functioning, substance abuse, immune dysfunction, cardiovascular illness, and suicide (Latham & Prigerson, 2004; Prigerson et al., 1997, 2009). Table 10.1 summarizes defining symptoms of CG. Clinicians should be alerted to these symptoms as they evaluate the longer-term adaptation of clients to the loss of a loved one, as both self-report (Keesee et al., 2008) and neurophysiological (O'Connor et al., 2008) data suggest that

TABLE 10.1
Diagnostic Features of Complicated Grief

1. Duration of bereavement of at least 6 months
2. Marked and persistent separation distress, reflected in intense feelings of loneliness, yearning for, or preoccupation with the person who has died
3. At least five of the following nine symptoms experienced nearly daily to a disabling degree:
    - Diminished sense of self (e.g., as if a part of oneself has died)
    - Difficulty accepting the loss on emotional as well as intellectual levels
    - Avoidance of reminders of the reality of the loss
    - Inability to trust others or to feel that others understand
    - Bitterness or anger over the death
    - Difficulty "moving on," or embracing new friends and interests
    - Numbness or inability to feel
    - Sensing that life or the future is without purpose or meaning
    - Feeling stunned, dazed, or shocked by the death
4. Significant impairment in social, occupational, or family functioning

Adapted from Prigerson et al. (2009) and Shear et al. (2011).

time alone does little to assuage CG symptomatology. Once identified, however, prolonged grief is clearly amenable to treatment (Shear et al., 2011).

RISK FACTORS FOR COMPLICATED GRIEF

Who is at risk for CG after a loss? To address this question, clinicians need to consider both fixed or relatively enduring characteristics of the survivor and shifting or circumstantial factors that bear on his or her ability to adapt to the death of a loved one. In the first category, each of us brings to loss aspects of ourselves such as gender, ethnicity, prior losses, attachment styles, and the role our deceased played in our lives (i.e., mother). Here, we will summarize our recent review of prospective risk factors for CG (Burke & Neimeyer, 2013), focusing on enduring individual differences associated with complications in bereavement. Following this, we will turn to circumstances of the death or treatment in the EOL period associated with poorer long-term outcomes for survivors, as well as factors observable in the course of bereavement that can become causes of concern, or alternatively suggest resilience in the wake of loss.

Predisposing Factors

Gender Differences

In terms of gender, Lang and Gottlieb (1993) found in their study of parents who had lost infants that mothers experienced higher levels of grief than did fathers. Likewise, although Spooren, Henderick, and Jannes (2000) found no difference in terms of the general psychological distress of 85 mothers and fathers bereaved by motor vehicle accidents (MVA), women did have higher levels of CG than did men. In a study of 151 Pakistani psychiatric patients, Prigerson et al. (2002) found that women had higher rates of CG than men, and, in a study of bereaved parents, Keesee et al. (2008) found that mothers had more grief than fathers but not more CG. Although gender differences are not always observed in bereavement adaptation, women tend to display greater susceptibility to separation distress than men.

Kinship Relation to the Deceased

Kinship (whether the deceased is one's spouse, parent, child, sibling, etc.) has been linked to intensified grief (Boelen, van den Bout, & van den Hout, 2003). For example, a large study ($N = 1,670$) with young adult grievers revealed a main effect for kinship in predicting CG, such that individuals bereft by the death of an immediate family member had higher grief than those who lost more distant family members (Laurie & Neimeyer, 2008). Likewise, Cleiren (1993) found that kinship remained the most powerful predictor of grief even 14 months post loss—spouses and parents suffered more in terms of grief than did adult children or siblings. And, consistently, mothers suffered most of all, even when controlling for other demographic factors. Similarly, Prigerson et al. (2002) compared types of relationships and found differences in CG levels, such that spouses and parents ($N = 151$) had much higher rates of CG than did other kinship types. Yet, other studies (Bonanno, Papa, Lalande, Zhang, & Noll, 2005) detected no initial differences until 14 months post loss, when parents' CG scores were higher than those of spouses.

Race and Ethnicity

Several studies have noted racial or ethnic differences in susceptibility to bereavement complication. Goldsmith and colleagues' (2008) two-sample study (316 bereaved individuals and 222 cancer patients and their caregivers), Laurie and Neimeyer's (2008) sample of 1,670 bereaved college students (940 Caucasians and 641 African Americans), and Neimeyer, Baldwin, and Gillies's (2006) study of 506 young adults all found higher levels of CG in African Americans than in Caucasians. Another study compared racial groups in a sample of 252 HIV-infected grievers and found that minorities (African Americans and Hispanics) reported more grief than Caucasians (Tarakeshwar, Hansen, Kochman, & Sikkema, 2005). However, a different study that examined race and CG in a sample of older, bereaved spouses found no difference in levels of yearning or grief when comparing African Americans ($n = 33$) and Caucasians ($n = 177$; Carr, 2004). Likewise, Cruz et al. (2007) found no differences among members of the same two ethnic groups presenting for CG therapy. Finally, in one of the rare international studies (Bonanno et al., 2005), research on bereaved parents ($n = 52$) and spouses ($n = 90$) from the People's Republic of China and the United States, assessed longitudinally at 4 and 18 months post loss, revealed that the Chinese sample had grief scores that were initially higher than those found in the U.S. sample, but later were lower than those of their American counterparts. In summary, many but not all studies of racial or ethnic differences in adaptation to bereavement suggest greater risk for ethnic minorities, at least within the United States, in keeping with broader research on mental health care disparities for different communities. Such findings shed little light, however, on factors that account for these disparities, underscoring the importance of studying cultural as well as individual factors that promote or impede adaptation (Rosenblatt & Wallace, 2005).

Attachment Styles

In research examining attachment styles, van der Houwen et al.'s (2010) study of 195 bereaved individuals indicated that avoidant but not anxious attachment signaled higher levels of CG. Brown, Neese, House, and Utz's (2009) study ($n = 103$) found at 6, 24, and 48 months that pre-loss insecure attachment style and post-loss grief were related. In two separate studies of 219 bereaved parents, Wijngaards-de Meij et al. (2007a, 2007b) found that avoidant/anxious attachment styles explained 13% of the variance in CG levels, and yet, other studies found no association between avoidant/dismissive attachment and grief (Bonanno et al., 2002).

Although more research is needed, a relation between the mourner's pre-loss dependency upon his or her spouse and subsequent grief also has been reported. Specifically, results from one study (Bonanno et al., 2002) prospectively linked pre-loss spousal dependency with CG, but not with resilience. Findings from another study (Carr, 2004), showed that spousal dependency predicted increased levels of grief-related despair. Yet, other studies show no such association (Cleiren, 1993).

Death-Related Risk Factors and EOL Considerations

Several studies (Gamino, Sewell, & Easterling, 2000; Rando, 1983) have linked the number of other losses experienced by the survivor with levels of grief. Post-loss bereavement can be influenced by pre-death factors such as quantity and quality of medical care, caregiver burden, acceptance of an anticipated death and/or anticipatory grieving, EOL decision making, one's religious or spiritual beliefs, how the death occurred (e.g., following a long illness vs. homicide), and other factors related to the final moments of life or shortly after (e.g., death notification).

Caregiver Burden, Acceptance, and Anticipatory Grief
The emotional and physical toll of caring for a dying loved one cannot be overstated, especially as it pertains to subsequent bereavement. In their six-wave longitudinal study of the impact of caregiving on depressive symptoms over time, Aneshensel, Botticello, and Yamamoto-Mitani (2004) found that caregiver burden significantly increased the probability of post-loss depressive symptoms and grief. Conversely, pre-death grief work can facilitate the mourning process. Examining data from 123 members of various online bereavement support groups, Metzger and Gray (2008) discovered that levels of pre-loss acceptance predicted less post-loss CG, even when time since loss and closeness to the deceased were held constant. However, this finding held true only in cases where grievers fully expected that their loved one would die. No such association was found between pre-loss acceptance and CG levels in survivors who did not foresee the death. McCarthy and associates conducted a study to examine rates of CG in 58 parents bereaved of a child to cancer (McCarthy et al., 2010). They found that rates of CG were predicted by less time since loss, preparedness for the death, economic hardship (as a result of the illness), and the parent's estimation of both the oncologist's care and the child's quality of life in his or her final days.

Moreover, research has shown that bereft individuals who have trouble adjusting to their loss in terms of grief may be less likely to have engaged in anticipatory grief behaviors (Rando, 1983). For example, Rando found in her study of 54 parents bereaved by their child's cancer that when anticipatory grieving was done prior to the death, less disordered grieving occurred afterward.

EOL Medical Care, Ethics, and Decision Making
One study of 332 caregivers who had lost their loved one on average 6 months prior found that aggressive medical intervention (e.g., admission to an intensive care unit, ventilation, resuscitation, chemotherapy, or use of a feeding tube) given to the patient prior to death predicted aspects of grief such as regret and feeling unprepared for the death (Wright et al., 2008).

From his review, Doka ascertained that EOL ethics and decisions can aid or prevent successful loss accommodation, sometimes simultaneously (Doka, 2005). Examples of instances where EOL decision making tended to predict CG included: terminating treatment or stopping heroic measures, family conflicts surrounding EOL care options, and torment related to the loved one's final moments (i.e., did he or she suffer needlessly due to thirst, starvation, or ineffective attempts at pain control). Ambivalence in itself has been found to increase grief, partly because it is so pervasive surrounding the death. For example, family members or caregivers may concomitantly wish for the loved one's suffering to end while at the same time wish to extend his or her life as long as possible (Doka, 2005). Similarly, it has been suggested that a highly ambivalent or poor pre-loss relationship between the deceased and survivor, where feelings were equally positive and negative, can intensify the post-loss grief reaction (Feigelman, Jordan, & Gorman, 2009; Worden, 2002).

Cause and Place of Death
Although exceptions exist (Prigerson et al., 2002), a growing body of studies indicates that violent death loss (e.g., homicide, suicide, or fatal accident) tends to elicit a more intense and complicated bereavement than deaths due to illness. For instance, in a study of Bosnian refugees, the strongest risk factor for CG occurred when one family member experienced the traumatic loss of another (Momartin, Silove, Manicavasagar, & Steel, 2004). Keesee et al. (2008) examined the full continuum of grief responses in a comparison study of parents bereaved as a result of violence and parents bereaved by other means, and found that violent death loss produced higher levels of grief. Other longitudinal studies comparing suicide and MVAs to extended illness (Cleiren, 1993), or survivors of illness to homicide, suicide, and accident (Gamino et al., 2000) found similar results—that violently bereaved individuals suffered more in terms of grief. Finally, in comparing type of death in 1,723 bereaved young adults, Currier, Holland, Coleman, and Neimeyer (2007) discovered that violent, unnatural death (accident, suicide, and homicide) was associated with worse bereavement outcome in terms of grief than death by other means (i.e., natural, anticipated deaths such as lengthy illness, or natural, sudden deaths such as heart attack). Although types of violent death loss (accident, suicide, or homicide) were not significantly different from one another, CG scores for survivors of violent death loss were significantly elevated over those of survivors of nonviolent loss; specifically, loss through homicide and accident was associated with more severe grief than was loss through sudden yet natural means (e.g., heart attack). Generally speaking, in comparison to all other types of death, homicide predicted poorer outcome in terms of grief.

In terms of where the death occurred, a study of 342 cancer caregivers whose loved one died in the hospital were 22% more susceptible to suffering from CG than caregivers whose loved one died at home under the care of hospice (Wright et al., 2010).

Peri-event Variables
Although research is limited, a consistent association has been found between peri-death factors and grief severity. One study of 210 suicide survivors found that although the method of suicide (e.g., gunshot) had little bearing on grief, finding or seeing the loved one's body immediately after the death significantly increased grief levels, especially for women (Callahan, 2000). Another comparison study of suicide survivors found that the greatest predictor of grief was finding the body immediately following the

death (Feigelman, Jordan, & Gorman, 2009), and, specifically, that elevated grief levels were more closely associated with grievers who saw or found the body than in survivors who had not seen the body following the suicide. Other studies (e.g., Spooren et al., 2000) have examined aspects surrounding MVA deaths of children, such as how and what the parents are told. They found that dissatisfaction with information given about the event and with material assistance predicted increased CG levels.

Religion and Spirituality

Prospective studies of the role of religion and spirituality in bereavement have produced mixed findings. For instance, one study showed that even though church attendance was unrelated, the greater importance placed on religious/spiritual beliefs before the loss meant that grievers had lower levels of grief at 6 and 18 months post loss (Brown et al., 2009). Other findings revealed the opposite, however. When 65 women who birthed a full-term baby were compared to 62 women who had terminated their pregnancy, individuals who valued their faith more experienced more severe grief than those who valued their faith less (Kersting et al., 2007). In their correlational study, Easterling et al. (2000) discovered an association between grievers' understanding of events that increase belief in God's existence and/or beliefs about their relationship with God and lower levels of grief. Other research (Bonanno et al., 2002) showed that individuals who fared best believed in a just world and were also more accepting of their loss.

Considering Mary's case in light of the pre-loss risk factors reviewed above, several features of her background, as well as features surrounding John's treatment and death, increased the probability of her responding to his loss with greater complication. These included (1) her gender, (2) her loss of her husband, (3) the threat this posed to a security-enhancing attachment, (4) her low acceptance of his prognosis, (5) his death in the relatively impersonal and technologically dominated hospital environment, and (6) the considerable ambivalence and conflict in the family regarding the course of his treatment. Table 10.2 provides a convenient checklist of risk factors for complicated or intensified grief observable before the death of a loved one, which in combination can help identify family members in need of heightened support during the EOL period.

Risk Factors in Bereavement

Factors subsequent to the loss itself, such as the amount of time since the death, quantity and quality of social support, beliefs about whether or not the death could have been prevented, the search for and success at meaning making, and other beliefs or fears about how well one is

TABLE 10.2
Pre-Loss Risk Factor Checklist for Complicated Grief
Research suggests that the following characteristics of the individual or family, the death itself, and the treatment context are associated with poorer adjustment in bereavement.

Background factors
✓Close kinship to the dying patient (especially spouse or child loss)
✓Female gender (especially mothers)
✓Minority ethnic status (in the United States)
✓Insecure attachment style
✓High pre-loss marital dependency

Death-related factors
✓Bereavement overload (multiple losses in quick succession)
✓Low acceptance of pending death
✓Violent death (suicide, homicide, accident)
✓Finding or viewing the loved one's body after violent death
✓Death in the hospital (vs. home)
✓Dissatisfaction with death notification

Treatment-related factors
✓Aggressive medical intervention (e.g., ICU, ventilation, resuscitation)
✓Ambivalence regarding treatment
✓Family conflict regarding treatment
✓Economic hardship created by treatment
✓Caregiver burden

doing or will fare in the days following have been shown to predict loss accommodation.

Initial Grief Responses

In their study comparing types of violent death loss, Feigelman et al. (2009) found that time since loss was the strongest predictor of grief difficulties, such that survivors who were most recently bereaved suffered the most. Survivors whose loved one died after a first-time suicide attempt rather than after a history of multiple attempts also suffered more grief.

Gamino et al. (2000) showed that bereaved individuals who maintained the belief that the death was preventable fared more poorly than those who did not. Doka (2005) echoed this, but also added that a lack of forewarning in terms of projecting that the death was imminent also prompted a more severe grief reaction.

Bereavement-associated Negative Cognitions

Boelen, van den Bout, and van den Hout (2006) measured early-bereavement thoughts (1–4 months post loss) that the griever held about his or her *self, life, future*, or *threatening interpretations of grief* (e.g., "If I would fully realize what the death of _ means, I would go crazy") and found that each individually predicted CG as bereavement progressed (7–10 months post loss). Moreover, negative cognitions specifically related to the *future* (e.g., "In the future, I will never become really happy anymore") prospectively predicted CG at the third assessment period, well over a year after the death (16–19 months post loss). The same held true in relation to an interaction effect of *threatening interpretations × avoidance of the reality of the loss* predicting CG at Time 3.

Searching for Meaning and Sense Making

Results of a prospective longitudinal study of older, bereaved adults (Coleman & Neimeyer, 2010) suggest that a more intense effort to find meaning in the loss was predictive of higher levels of grief. Even 4 years after the death, grievers who could not make sense of the loss early on (6 and 18 months post loss) still struggled with high grief distress. In contrast, those who could find a way to make sense of their loss experienced a greater sense of overall well-being—showing interest and excitement in life, and a sense of personal accomplishment (see also Davis, Wortman, Lehman, & Silver, 2000). Importantly, high separation distress early in bereavement also prospectively predicted spiritual struggle, suggesting that a vicious circle can be set in motion in which intense grief can exacerbate problems with spiritual sense making in the wake of loss (Burke, Neimeyer, McDevitt-Murphy, Ippolito, & Roberts, 2011).

Social Support

Rando (1983) showed that bereaved parents with greater amounts of support suffered less grief. Laurie and Neimeyer (2008) found in their comparison study of young-adult grievers that African Americans spent less time talking about their losses than did Caucasians and that less time discussing the loss was associated with increased grief scores. Identification of modifiable risk factors, such as social support, can guide the development of relevant secondary or tertiary interventions. For instance, armed with the knowledge that poor social support (i.e., negative interactions) poses risks to bereavement adaptation (Burke, Neimeyer, & McDevitt-Murphy, 2010), health care professionals in EOL contexts could assess families' social support before bereavement begins, with an eye toward preventive intervention.

Mary's case exemplifies most of these features associated with intense and prolonged grief reactions, including (1) strong initial responses to her husband's death; (2) little warning of his death given the brief period since his diagnosis; (3) her sense that the death could have been prevented by earlier detection of his symptoms; (4) her fatalism regarding the purposelessness and joylessness of a future without John; (5) her avoidance of the reality of his death, as in her insistence in washing his clothes repeatedly, as if he were merely away on a trip; (6) her anguished search for meaning and struggle with God's intentions in taking his life; and (7) the low social support she experienced as a function of withdrawing from many relationships and isolating herself in her grief. Clinical Pearl 10.1 provides a convenient list of factors observable in bereavement that predict more intense and prolonged grieving for survivors, and associated principles to guide intervention.

CLINICAL PEARL

Areas of Concern in Bereavement and Associated Principles of Intervention

Early responses to death

- *Initial grief responses are most intense*, and call for immediate support, though not necessarily formal therapy.
- *Lack of warning regarding the death forecasts more severe bereavement distress*, which can be mitigated by keeping families fully and honestly informed regarding their loved one's changing condition.
- *Perception that the death was preventable predicts more intense grief*, suggesting a role for realistic assurance that the family and medical team did all that could reasonably be done to preserve the patient's life.

Cognitive and behavioral factors

- *Negative interpretations of the self, world, and future in the wake of loss are associated with more complicated grief*, and could be indications for professional therapy if self-criticism or fatalism becomes entrenched.
- *Avoidance of the reality of the loss impedes adaptation*, highlights the relevance of interventions that involve review of the narrative of the loss using compassionate witnessing and support, and requires collaboration in sorting through its implications for survivors.
- *An anguished search for meaning in the loss that finds no answers forecasts protracted grief*, and calls for spiritual or secular counsel to help survivors make sense of the death and find changed significance in their ongoing lives.
- *Low social support and negative, critical, or intrusive interactions exacerbate grief*, and call for provision of temporary support (e.g., in survivors groups) as well as possible therapy to promote skillful management of other relationships in the family or community.

AVAILABLE TREATMENTS FOR BEREAVED INDIVIDUALS

Grieving is the natural, normal, and often necessary response of humans to loss. Thus, professional treatment is not always required, as most bereaved individuals adapt well over time, given their own resources and those of their families and communities. However, when grief is complicated and prolonged, evidence suggests that intervention is both indicated and efficacious (Currier, Neimeyer, & Berman, 2008). Fortunately, several research-informed treatments exist, both for use prior to the loss and afterward. The following are examples of grief-specific interventions.

Family focused grief therapy (FFGT; Kissane & Bloch, 2002). FFGT is a pre-loss intervention that screens "at risk" families into the intervention that spans 6 to 18 months, beginning several months before the loved one dies and continuing through bereavement for 6 to 12 sessions, depending upon the family's distress level. Based on the family relationships index (FRI), families are classified as either well-functioning (i.e., *supportive*—showing a high level of cohesion, or *conflict resolving*—permitting and accepting each others' differences and dealing with discord constructively) or dysfunctional (*hostile*—families characterized by high conflict, low cohesion, and poor expressiveness, or *sullen*—families characterized by poor communication, depression, and muted anger). A final *intermediate* group shows some impairment in communication and teamwork, although conflict is less intense than in the hostile group (Kissane & Hooghe, 2011). According to Kissane and Zaider (2011), over half of the families of dying cancer patients are well-functioning and thus do not need therapy; however, immediately following the death, approximately 20% of families fall into the dysfunctional categories and are in need of specialized therapeutic attention. Importantly, however, Kissane and Bloch (2002) have also found that although sullen and intermediate families respond well to family therapy, hostile families do not, and instead deteriorate in conjoint sessions. For this reason, the latter families, marked by stormy and unresolved conflict, are better offered individual treatment, where each member's unique needs can be assessed and addressed without the compounded distress generated by family sessions.

Kissane and Bloch (2002) outlined a number of key therapeutic processes and challenges inherent to the family engaged in FFGT, including inviting a discussion of death into the room, by speaking candidly about the illness and its prognosis. Specifically, therapists are urged to: (1) encourage families to view the loss in hypothetical rather than impending terms, and (2) maintain a neutral stance when it comes to juxtaposing hopeful family members with those who are already experiencing anticipatory grief reactions. Preserving an impartial position enables the clinician to serve the family dispassionately in spite of their discrepant coping styles. Other families will need the therapist's active involvement for them to engage in conversation at all—even to the point of the therapist inviting each member individually. Likewise, therapy conducted in the home must by necessity include clear boundaries in order to establish a therapeutic environment minus the distraction caused by TV, phone calls, and other factors. In addition, cross-cultural challenges surface when individual members with distinct expectations about the dying process attempt to mesh as a family unit. Thus, prior to death, the clinician may invite the family to decide together exactly what, how, and how much they will discuss. Families with young children bereft of a parent might need special attention. Kissane and Zaider (2011) and Kissane and Hooghe (2011) claim that when a model that encourages candid expression of thoughts and feelings is used, it also strengthens the surviving parent's belief that he or she can manage as a single parent. However, great sensitivity is advised in pursuing such conversations, respecting the wisdom of both talking and *not talking*, a means of regulating difficult emotions within and between family members (Kissane & Hooghe, 2011). Clinical Pearl 10.2 summarizes several of these recommendations for clinical practice.

CLINICAL PEARL

Principles of Family Therapy Near the EOL

EOL issues pose challenges for both families and clinicians engaged in the pre-loss therapeutic processes. In family focused grief therapy (FFGT; Kissane & Bloch, 2002), the process includes family members talking with each other about the illness and about their future needs, problems with engaging family members, limits to therapeutic goals, therapy in the home, cross-cultural challenges, working with families with young children, and ethical issues.

EOL discussions

- *Talking about the illness and prognosis,* forthrightly, is easier for some family members if addressed speculatively rather than definitively, and if room is given to both those who maintain hope for positive progress and those who have already begun the grieving process.
- *Discussions about future needs,* once the loved one has died, are facilitated by future-oriented questions that identify anticipated needs and outline a proactive plan for engaging support.

Therapy challenges

- *Engaging family members in conversation* is most difficult in families with minimal cohesion, requiring extra involvement on the part of the clinician.

(continued)

CLINICAL PEARL (continued)

- *Limits to therapy goals* exist in the face of the myriad pre-illness and ongoing stressors facing even the most intact families.
- *Home therapy* occurring alongside hospice care may not suit every family, and requires the establishment of boundaries in order to prevent barriers to therapy.
- *Cross-cultural issues* surrounding death rituals and EOL mores can cause unnecessary family stress unless addressed openly, with respect for differing views.
- *Young children* in a family anticipating a parent's death require special consideration to facilitate a healthy grieving process, which, in turn, can bolster the confidence and skills of the surviving parent.
- *Maintaining an "ethic of care"* is the basis of FFGT, with preference and sensitivity shown to various family members in need of special attention at a given point in the dying and grieving process.

Complicated grief treatment (CGT; Shear, Frank, Houch, & Reynolds, 2005) is an individual intervention specifically designed to address CG symptoms in bereaved individuals. It consists of 10 modules that include psychoeducation about grief work, as well as experientially powerful engagement with one's own distress over the loss. *Imaginal revisiting* of the story of the death, in which the griever verbally shares his or her detailed account of the death event from the moment of notification until the burial, is a key component of CGT. Such revisiting typically elevates the survivor's initial distress level considerably, with the goal of promoting mastery of the distressing experience in the compassionate presence of the therapist. Similarly, *situational revisiting* challenges behaviors and cognitions that reinforce the perpetual avoidance of places, people, or events that cause the griever significant distress in bereavement but were once enjoyed freely, thereby promoting fuller engagement with life. CGT also includes *imaginal conversation* between the client and the deceased, with the therapist helping the client to participate in a two-way symbolic conversation with the deceased loved one to resolve troubling concerns that haunt the relationship, such as caregiver guilt arising from the circumstances of the death. Additional modules of the therapy tap into both positive and negative memories that the survivor has in relation to the deceased loved one, in what is referred to as *emotional memory work*, and helps him or her to revise life goals and meaningful relationships as he or she engages in *future planning*. Although CGT is principally an individual intervention, it also commonly includes inviting a trusted family member or friend to join the client and therapist in one or more sessions as a means of showing support of CGT for the griever (Shear, Boelen, & Neimeyer, 2011; Shear, Gorscak, & Simon,

2006). To test the efficacy of this multicomponent intervention, Shear and her team (2005) conducted a randomized control trial with 95 grievers, comparing it to interpersonal psychotherapy (IPT), an evidence-based treatment that has been found efficacious for treating depression. CGT reduced the incidence of CG by 51%, compared to 28% for IPT, and was particularly efficacious for those suffering violent death loss.

Cognitive behavioral therapy (CBT) for CG (Boelen, van den Hout, & van den Bout, 2006) is grounded in the assumption that grievers need to integrate the loss into their existing autobiographical knowledge, change patterns of thinking that are unhelpful, and replace unhelpful avoidance strategies with helpful actions and coping strategies. As with CGT, one important component of CBT is *exposure*. Clients may narrate their loss experience in verbal or written form, expressing the most difficult and painful aspects of the death. Subsequently, grievers are instructed to cease behaviors that are considered compulsive (e.g., asking "why" the death happened, visiting the gravesite). Related CBT strategies include confrontation of anxious avoidance of people, situations, and thoughts based on predictions that the pain of the loss in some way will be too much to endure, so as to build more adaptive behaviors.

A second component of CBT is *cognitive restructuring*—the systematic identification and reorganization of one's thoughts, and the substitution of unhelpful cognitions with helpful ones. For example, hopeless statements about one's future might be challenged with, "What might be the outcome of maintaining the expectation that you will never be happy again?" Likewise, in learning, for instance, that the bereaved person's social network is steadily withdrawing from him or her, the therapist might encourage the individual to specifically set up a time to discuss this topic openly with family or friends and engage in corrective action.

Using exposure and cognitive restructuring techniques, therapists help clients face internal and external stimuli in order to learn that tolerating loss-related distress is possible and that ultimately it lessens suffering rather than increases it. Similarly, clinicians can employ behavioral activation to target depressive avoidance that may have prevented the survivor from engaging in pleasurable activities. Primarily, this is accomplished by encouraging the client to engage in gratifying activities even before he or she senses an intrinsic ability to do so. As Boelen et al. (2006) aptly argued, "action often precedes mood improvement and adjustment" (p. 111). A randomized, controlled trial of CBT for CG demonstrates that it outperforms supportive counseling, and suggests that exposure interventions may be especially effective (Boelen, de Keijser, van den Hout, & van den Bout, 2007).

Meaning reconstruction approaches to grief therapy (Neimeyer, 2000) posit that grieving entails an active effort to reaffirm or reconstruct a world of meaning that has been challenged by loss. In this perspective, people are viewed as meaning makers, drawing on personal and cultural resources to construct a system of beliefs that permit them to anticipate and respond to the essential events of their lives. The life-threatening illness and death of a loved one, however, can challenge this framework, sometimes calling into question the central themes of a person's worldview and self-narrative, or life story, across time. Such a perspective accords well with a growing body of research that points to the anguished search for meaning into which the bereaved are frequently cast, and the tendency for enhanced sense making in the wake of such tragic losses to be associated with more favorable bereavement outcomes (Neimeyer & Sands, 2011).

Accordingly, therapeutic efforts concentrate on two key domains of meaning reconstruction, through assisting the bereaved individual to process the *event story* of the death as well as to access and reconstruct attachment security in the *back story* of his or her relationship to the deceased (Neimeyer, 2011). For example, following careful cultivation of an empathic presence to the mourner's pain, the therapist can support him or her in retelling the narrative of the loss, with emphasis on those occurrences that were particularly distressing and likely to be "edited out" of the accounts shared with others. Tracking back and forth between the external, objective story of what transpired and associated internal feelings and emotions, the therapist is vigilant for unanswered questions and troubling meanings implied by the account, and joins the client in seeking more sustainable answers. Likewise, the therapist joins the client in the characteristic quest to not so much relinquish attachment to the deceased, but to reconstruct it in a form that does not require his or her physical presence in the client's life. For example, the therapist may use any number of experientially vivid techniques to invoke the presence of the deceased in therapy (e.g., through a review of photos or mementos, symbolically corresponding with the deceased or facilitating conversations between the deceased and the bereaved, with the latter loaning the former his or her voice to reanimate their dialogue).

A distinctive feature of this constructivist approach is the use of creative writing to promote both review of the event story of the death in a way that promotes sense making and benefit finding in the experience, and accessing the ongoing relationship with and legacy of the deceased as a source of security and continued orientation in living. Such techniques have found support in randomized, controlled studies of writing interventions that foster meaning making and perspective taking in the wake of loss, both in conventional written (Lichtenthal & Cruess, 2010) and Internet-administered (Wagner, Knaevelsrud, & Maercker, 2006) forms. A representative set of methods for promoting meaning reconstruction appears in Table 10.3, and detailed instructions for several of these methods have been provided elsewhere (Neimeyer, 2012). Video demonstrations of meaning reconstruction in actual cases of grief therapy are also available (Neimeyer, 2004, 2008).

TABLE 10.3
Techniques for Facilitating Meaning Reconstruction in Bereavement

As bereavement typically challenges mourners to contend with the significance of the loss as well as to reconstruct their relationship to the deceased, meaning-centered therapy incorporates a variety of procedures for promoting both outcomes. The following representative sample of techniques is derived from the manual of creative practices for grief therapy compiled by Neimeyer (2012), which provides detailed instructions for each, illustrated by case studies.

Processing and Integrating the Event Story of the Death

Retelling the narrative of the death	Slow-motion review of the loss story to promote mastery
Loss timelines	Situating the current loss in the landscape of previous experience
Virtual dream stories	Creative writing about loss themes to facilitate their exploration
Playing with playlists	Tracing the trajectory of love and loss in musical memoir on iPod
Figurative sand tray therapy	Constructing symbolic stories using figurines in sand world
Analogical listening	Focusing on bodily felt sense of grief and giving it expression
The body of trust	Depicting impact of the death story in mixed media on body image
Directed journaling	Diary work to consolidate sense making and benefit finding
Loss characterization	Narrating overall impact of loss on one's sense of self
Overt statements	Voicing deep meanings that make chronic grief necessary
Rituals of transition	Symbolically validating life changes occasioned by loss

Accessing and Reconstructing the Back Story of the Relationship to the Deceased

Introducing the deceased	Reclaiming the deceased as a participant in one's ongoing life
Imaginal conversations	Visualizing the deceased while addressing unfinished business
Correspondence with the deceased	Inviting an "exchange" of letters to renegotiate the relationship
Chair work	Choreographing deeply authentic conversation with the deceased
Life imprint	Tracing the impact of the deceased on one's values and decisions
Reviewing the photo album	Consolidating memories with the therapist as a witness
Prescriptive photomontage	Constructing creative composite image of deceased's role in life
Memory books and boxes	Organizing mementos and messages that honor legacy of the lost
Rituals of connection	Symbolically validating continuing bonds

CASE 2: AN ILLUSTRATIVE CASE STUDY

Kenya's pursuit of therapy (with the first author) was prompted by a number of recent but frightening physical symptoms, which included dizziness, rapid heartbeat, and racing pulse, accompanied by general sadness and spiritual malaise. When thorough medical testing disclosed no organic basis for these reactions, her physician referred her for psychotherapy with a diagnosis of "panic attacks of psychogenic origin" as well as possible depression, which had been unresponsive to medication. Presenting for her first session attractively attired in a conservative suit, Kenya noted that her symptoms worsened when she prepared to leave the northern city that had been "her only home" some 5 months earlier to follow her husband's "call" to take a position as the pastor of a southern African American church over a thousand miles away. Now, distant from her mother, sisters, and friends in the community that had shaped and sustained her, she found herself becoming increasingly reclusive, lest members of the new congregation discover her "emotional problems" and label her as "crazy." Over the past several weeks, Kenya confided, she had begun to "pull away" from her husband, George, and 12-year-old daughter, Leitha, deepening her concern that she not only was failing as the "first lady" of her church, but also was "losing herself" and those she loved.

After exploring Kenya's understanding of her problem in more detail, I inquired about any previous experiences she might have had with therapy, and learned that she had briefly sought counseling following her father's death a few years before, the stress of which had been compounded by the long illness that preceded it, and for which she and her mother had been the primary caregivers. Tears rolled down Kenya's cheeks in response to my empathic inquiry about the trembling in her lip as she recounted her father's passing, and she noted that she had only in the past year begun to cry for him, as his uncharacteristic "meanness" during his illness and treatment left her with a complex blend of avoidance and grief over his passing. Now, she realized, she keenly felt the separation from him, and, speaking quietly through a haze of tears, added that, "He would have been able to give me advice about moving, if only he were here."

Alerted to the emotional vividness of this material for Kenya years after her father's death, and struck by her spontaneous linkage of his absence with the problems in her relocation, I gently asked Kenya if she would like to invite her father to join us in the therapy room, to reopen a relationship with him that had been interrupted by his illness and death. Intrigued, she accepted the suggestion, and with guidance began a conversation with her father, who we symbolically offered an empty chair positioned across from his daughter. Sobbing, Kenya recounted to her father the outlines of her current problems, and, after a few seconds of silence, deepened her disclosure to include her feeling of guilt for having "abandoned" him by leaving the city in which he had lived for his whole adult life, to move to the South he had known only as a boy.

Accepting my suggestion that she take her father's place and respond to what she had said, Kenya changed chairs, dried her tears, and offered reassurance, concluding with, "Don't worry, Baby, I'll come visit you," words that rung strangely hollow in view of the poignant sense of loss that Kenya had shared only moments before. Again taking her own seat at my gesture, Kenya repeated the words I tentatively offered to her: "You can't visit me, Dad. You're dead." Kenya then poured forth both her grief and self-doubt, punctuated by wracking sobs. As she grew quiet, I again invited her into her father's chair, where, unprompted, Kenya (as her father) provided loving and genuine reassurance, affirming that, despite his death, he would always be with her spiritually and emotionally, always believe in her. This interaction triggered a startling insight for Kenya. In her words, "I realize now that I *can* keep him, that he *can* be with me, and that I can even come to know him more through the South that he loved." Buoyed up by the newfound reconnection with her father, Kenya then went on to consider her own sense of being uprooted from the surviving members of her family of origin, who, like her, were "struggling together to make sense of this new transition." As our first session ended, Kenya somewhat sheepishly shared her wish to pursue advanced schooling, despite her "first lady" status. However, serving as a cultural interpreter, she described for my benefit as a Caucasian therapist the implicit social expectations within some African American faith communities that constrained this potentially "selfish" goal. Eager to pursue the "fresh ideas" generated in the session, Kenya closed by requesting another appointment.

In her remaining three bi-weekly sessions, Kenya deepened her exploration of both her history of loss, revisiting the story of the death of an infant son early in her marriage, and renewed her effort to "find her own voice" as a woman in her family and church community. As she did so, she remarked with some surprise that life was starting to seem somehow "more real," and she related with pride several concrete instances in which she had negotiated important family decisions with her husband, played a more active role in providing guidance to her pre-teen daughter, and "stood up" for innovative programs she advocated in the church. In all of this, she continued to experience a strong sense of her father's presence and pride in her, and the feeling that something had "lifted" for her in the pivotal "conversation" with him in the opening session. In Kenya's own words, she no longer felt "held back," and was gratified by George's support for her being her own "outspoken" self, even to the point of wearing neat, yet more casual clothes to both church committee meetings and therapy sessions. Perhaps most remarkably, she had been entirely freed of the panic symptoms from the point of her "conversation" with her father onward, despite these symptoms never having been made the specific targets of therapeutic intervention. Our therapy concluded by reflecting on the "changed narrative" of Kenya's life, which re-established a meaningful sense of continuity with whom she had been (as anchored in an ongoing relationship with her supportive father), while also permitting her to "re-author" aspects of her identity in critical living relationships. Follow-up indicated that these changes were consolidated over the months to come.

CONCLUSION

Loss may be inevitable in human life, but the experience of intense, protracted grieving is not. In this chapter we have summarized the features and risk factors for complicated grief, both in the context of EOL care and in subsequent bereavement, and attempted to offer some principles for mitigating the suffering of survivors. When these efforts to assist family members whose loved ones are dying are supplemented with therapies for those whose grief seems unresponsive to the passage of time, there is reason to hope that the bereaved can find their way from mourning to meaning, so that their own lives are strengthened through a containing bond with their loved one (Klass, Silverman, & Nickman, 1996) rather than damaged by loss.

REFERENCES

Aneshensel, C. S., Botticello, A. L., & Yamamoto-Mitani, N. (2004). When caregiving ends: The course of depressive symptoms after bereavement. *Journal of Health and Social Behavior, 45,* 422–440.

Boelen, P., van den Hout, M., & van den Bout, J. (2006). A cognitive-behavioral conceptualization of complicated grief. *Clinical Psychology: Science and Practice, i*(13), 109–128.

Boelen, P. A., de Keijser, J., van den Hout, M., & van den Bout, J. (2007). Treatment of complicated grief: A comparison between cognitive-behavioral therapy and supportive counseling. *Journal of Clinical and Consulting Psychology, 75,* 277–284.

Boelen, P. A., & Prigerson, H. G. (2007). The influence of symptoms of prolonged grief disorder, depression, and anxiety on quality of life bereaved adults: A prospective study. *European Archives of Psychiatry and Clinical Neuroscience, 257,* 444–452.

Boelen, P. A., van den Bout, J., & van den Hout, M. A. (2003). The role of negative interpretations of grief reactions in emotional problems after bereavement. *Journal of Behavior Therapy and Experimental Psychiatry, 34,* 225–238.

Bonanno, G. A., & Kaltman, S. (2001). The varieties of grief experience. *Clinical Psychology Review, 21,* 705–734.

Bonanno, G. A., Papa, A., Lalande, K., Zhang, N., & Noll, J. G. (2005). Grief processing and deliberate grief avoidance: A prospective comparison of bereaved spouses

and parents in the United States and the Peoples Republic of China. *Journal of Counseling and Clinical Psychology, 73,* 86–98.
Bonanno, G. A., Wortman, C. B., Lehman, D. R., Tweed, R. G., Haring, M., Sonnega, J. et al. (2002). Resilience to loss and chronic grief. *Journal of Personality and Social Psychology, 83,* 1150–1164.
Bonanno, G. A., Wortman, C. B., & Nesse, R. M. (2004). Prospective patterns of resilience and maladjustment during widowhood. *Psychology and Aging, 19,* 260–271.
Brown, S. L., Nesse, R. M., House, J. S., & Utz, R. L. (2009). Religion and emotional compensation: Results from a prospective study of widowhood. *Society for Personality and Social Psychology, 30,* 1165–1174.
Burke, L. A., & Neimeyer, R. A. (2013). Prospective risk factors for complicated grief: A review of the empirical literature. In M. Stroebe, H. Schut, P. Boelen, & J. van den Bout (Eds.), *Complicated grief: Scientific foundations for health care professionals.* (pp. 145–161). Washington, DC: American Psychological Association.
Burke, L. A., Neimeyer, R. A., & McDevitt-Murphy, M. E. (2010). African American homicide bereavement: Aspects of social support that predict complicated grief, PTSD and depression. *Omega, 61,* 1–24.
Burke, L. A., Neimeyer, R. A., McDevitt-Murphy, M. E., Ippolito, M. R., & Roberts, J. M. (2011). In the wake of homicide: Spiritual crisis and bereavement distress in an African American sample. *International Journal Psychology of Religion, 21,* 1–19. doi: 10.1080/10508619.2011.60741.
Callahan, J. (2000). Predictors and correlates of bereavement in suicide support group participants. *Suicide and Life Threatening Behavior, 30,* 104–124.
Carr, D. S. (2004). African American/Caucasian differences in psychological adjustment to spousal loss among older adults. *Research on Aging, 26,* 591–622.
Cleiren, M. (1993). *Bereavement and adaptation: A comparative study of the aftermath of death.* Washington, DC: Hemisphere Publishing Co.
Coleman, R. A., & Neimeyer, R. A. (2010). Measuring meaning: Searching for and making sense of spousal loss in later life. *Death Studies, 34,* 804–834.
Cruz, M., Scott, J., Houck, P., Reynolds, C. F., III., Frank, E., & Shear, M. K. (2007). Cinical presentation and treatment outcome of African Americans with complicated grief. *Psychiatric Services, 58,* 700–702.
Currier, J. M., Holland, J., Coleman, R., & Neimeyer, R. A. (2007). Bereavement following violent death: An assault on life and meaning. In R. Stevenson & G. Cox (Eds.), *Perspectives on violence and violent death* (pp. 175–200). Amityville, NY: Baywood.
Currier, J. M., Neimeyer, R. A., & Berman, J. S. (2008). The effectiveness of psychotherapeutic interventions for the bereaved: A comprehensive quantitative review. *Psychological Bulletin, 134,* 648–661.
Davis, C. G., Wortman, C. B., Lehman, D. R., & Silver, R. C. (2000). Searching for meaning in loss: Are clinical assumptions correct? *Death Studies, 24,* 497–540.
Doka, K. J. (2005). Ethics, end-of-life decisions and grief. *Mortality, 10*(1), 83–90. doi: 10.1080/1357627500031105.
Easterling, L. W., Gamino, L. A., Sewell, K. W., & Stirman, L. S. (2000). Spiritual experience, church attendance, and bereavement. *Journal of Pastoral Care, 54,* 263–275.

Feigelman, W., Jordan, J. R., & Gorman, B. S. (2009). How they died, time since loss, and bereavement outcomes. *Omega: Journal of Death and Dying, 58*, 251–273.

Gamino, L. A., Sewell, K. W., & Easterling, L. W. (2000). Scott and White grief study phase 2: Toward an adaptive model of grief. *Death Studies, 24*, 633–660.

Goldsmith, B., Morrison, R. S., Vanderwerker, L. C., & Prigerson, H. (2008). Elevated rates of prolonged grief disorder in African Americans. *Death Studies, 32*, 352–365.

Holland, J. M., Neimeyer, R. A., Boelen, P. A., & Prigerson, H. G. (2009). The underlying structure of grief: A taxometric investigation of prolonged and normal reactions to loss. *Journal of Psychopathology and Behavioral Assessment, 31*, 190–201.

Keesee, N. J., Currier, J. M., & Neimeyer, R. A. (2008). Predictors of grief following the death of one's child: The contribution of finding meaning. *Journal of Clinical Psychology, 64*, 1–19.

Kersting, A., Kroker, K., Steinhard, J., Ludorff, K., Wesselmann, U., & Ohrmann, P. (2007). Complicated grief after traumatic loss: A 14-month follow-up study. *European Archive of Psychiatry Clinical Neuroscience, 257*, 437–443.

Kissane, D. W., & Bloch, S. (2002). *Family focused grief therapy: A model of family-centered care during palliative care and bereavement.* Buckingham, UK: Open University Press.

Kissane, D. W., & Hooghe, A. (2011). Family therapy for the bereaved. In R. A. Neimeyer, D. L. Harris, H. R. Winokuer, & G. F. Thornton (Eds.), *Grief and bereavement in contemporary society: Bridging research and practice* (pp. 287–302). New York, NY: Routledge.

Kissane, D. W., & Zaider, T. I. (2011). Family Focused therapy in palliative care and bereavement. In M. Watson, & D. Kissane (Eds.), *Handbook of psychotherapy in cancer care* (pp. 185–197). New York City: Wiley-Blackwell.

Klass, D., Silverman, P. R., & Nickman, S. L. (1996). *Continuing bonds: New understandings of grief.* Levittown, PA: Taylor & Francis.

Lang, A., & Gottlieb, L. (1993). Parental grief reactions and marital intimacy following infant death. *Death Studies, 17*, 233–255.

Latham, A., & Prigerson, H. (2004). Suicidality and bereavement: Complicated grief as psychiatric disorder presenting greatest risk for suicidality. *Suicide and Life Threatening Behavior, 34*, 350–362.

Laurie, A., & Neimeyer, R. A. (2008). African Americans and bereavement: Grief as a function of ethnicity. *Omega, 57*, 173–193.

Lichtenthal, W. G., & Cruess, D. G. (2010). Effects of directed written disclosure on grief and distress symptoms among bereaved individuals. *Death Studies, 34*, 475–499.

McCarthy, M. C., Clarke, N. E., Ting, C. L., Conroy, R., Anderson, V. A., & Heath, J. A. (2010). Prevalence and predictors of parental grief and depression after the death of a child from cancer. *Journal of Palliative Medicine, 13*(11), 1321–1326. doi: 10.1089/jpm.2010.0037.

McDaid, C., Trowman, R., Golder, S., Hawton, K., & Sowden, A. (2008). Interventions for people bereaved through suicide: Systematic review. *The British Journal of Psychiatry, 193*, 438–443.

McDevitt-Murphy, M. E., Neimeyer, R. A., Burke, L. A., & Williams, J. L. (2012). Assessing the toll of traumatic loss: Psychological symptoms in African Americans bereaved by homicide. *Psychological Trauma, 4*(3), 303–311.

Metzger, P. L., & Gray, M. J. (2008). End-of-life communication and adjustment: Pre-loss communication as a predictor of bereavement-related outcomes. *Death Studies, 32*, 301–325. doi: 10.1080/07481180801928923.

Momartin, S., Silove, D., Manicavasagar, V., & Steel, Z. (2004). Complicated grief in Bosnian refugees: Associations with posttraumatic stress disorder and depression. *Comprehensive Psychiatry, 45*, 475–482.

Neimeyer, R. A. (2000). Searching for the meaning of meaning: Grief therapy and the process of reconstruction. *Death Studies, 24*, 541–558.

Neimeyer, R. A. (2004). Constructivist psychotherapy. *Series 1: Systems of psychotherapy* [VHS video/DVD]. Washington, DC: American Psychological Association.

Neimeyer, R. A. (2008). *Constructivist psychotherapy over time* [DVD]. Washington, DC: American Psychological Association.

Neimeyer, R. A. (2011). Reconstructing meaning in bereavement. In M. W. D. Kissane (Ed.), *Handbook of psychotherapy in cancer care* (pp. 247–257). New York City: Wiley-Blackwell.

Neimeyer, R. A. (2012). *Techniques in grief therapy: Creative strategies for counseling the bereaved*. New York: Routledge.

Neimeyer, R. A., Baldwin, S. A., & Gillies, J. (2006). Continuing bonds and reconstructing meaning: Mitigating complications in bereavement. *Death Studies, 30*, 715–738.

Neimeyer, R. A., & Sands, D. C. (2011). Meaning reconstruction in bereavement: From principles to practice. In R. A. Neimeyer, H. Winokuer, D. Harris, & G. Thornton (Eds.), *Grief and bereavement in contemporary society: Bridging research and practice.* (pp. 9–22). New York: Routledge.

O' Connor, M. F., Wellisch, D. K., Stanton, A. L., Eisenberger, N. I., Irwin, M. R., & Lieberman, M. D. (2008). Craving love? Enduring grief activates brain's reward center. *Neuro Image, 42*, 969–972.

Prigerson, H., Ahmed, I., Silverman, G. K., Saxena, A. K., Maciejewski, P. K., Jacobs, S. C., ... Hamirani, M. (2002). Rates of risks of complicated grief among psychiatric clinic patients in Karachi Pakistan. *Death Studies, 26*, 781–792.

Prigerson, H. G., Beirhals, A. J., Kasl, S. V., Reynolds, C. F., 3rd, Shear, M. K., Day, H., ... Jacobs, S. (1997). Traumatic grief as a risk factor for mental and physical morbidity. *American Journal of Psychiatry, 154*, 616–623.

Prigerson, H. G., Frank, E., Kasl, S., Reynolds, C., Anderson, B., Zubenko, G. S., ... Kupfer, D. J. (1995). Complicated grief and bereavement related depression as distinct disorders: Preliminary empirical validation in elderly bereaved spouses. *American Journal of Psychiatry, 152*, 22–30.

Prigerson, H. G., Horowitz, M. J., Jacobs, S. C., Parkes, C. M., Aslan, M., Goodkin, K., Raphael, B., ... Maciejewski, P. K. (2009). Prolonged grief disorder: Psychometric validation of criteria proposed for DSM-V and ICD-11. *PLoS Medicine, 6*(8), 1–12.

Prigerson, H. G., & Jacobs, S. C. (2001). Traumatic grief as a distinct disorder: A rationale, consensus criteria, and a preliminary empirical test. In M. S. Stroebe, R. O. Hansson, W. Stroebe, & H. Schut (Eds.), *Handbook of bereavement research* (pp. 613–645). Washington, DC: American Psychological Association.

Rando, T. A. (1983). An investigation of grief and adaptation in parents whose children have died from cancer. *Journal of Pediatric Psychology, 8*(1), 3–20.

Rosenblatt, P., & Wallace, B. (2005). *African American grief*. New York: Routledge.

Shear, K., Boelen, P., & Neimeyer, R. A. (2011). Treating complicated grief: Converging approaches. In R. A. Neimeyer, D. Harris, H. Winokuer, & G. Thornton (Eds.), *Grief and bereavement in contemporary society: Bridging research and practice* (pp. 139–162). New York: Routledge.

Shear, K., Frank, E., Houch, P. R., & Reynolds, C. F. (2005). Treatment of complicated grief: A randomized controlled trial. *Journal of the American Medical Association, 293,* 2601–2608.

Shear, K., Gorscak, B., & Simon, N. (2006). Treatment of complicated grief following violet death. In E. K. Rynearson (Ed.), *Violent death: Reslience and intervention beyond the crisis* (pp. 157–174). New York: Routledge.

Shear, M. K., Jackson, C. T., Essock, S. M., Donahue, S. A., & Felton, C. J. (2006). Screening for complicated grief among Project Liberty service recipients 18 months after September 11, 2001. *Psychiatric Services, 57,* 1291–1297.

Shear, M. K., Simon, N., Wall, M., Zisook, S., Neimeyer, R., Duan, N., . . . Keshaviah, A. (2011). Complicated grief and related bereavement issues for DSM-5. *Depression and Anxiety, 28*(2), 103–117. doi: 10.1002/da.20780.

Spooren, D. J., Henderick, H., & Jannes, C. (2000). Survey description of stress of parents bereaved from a child killed in a traffic accident: A retrospective study of a victim support group. *Omega: Journal of Death and Dying, 42,* 171–185.

Stroebe, M., Schut, H., & Stroebe, W. (2007). Health outcomes in bereavement. *Lancet, 370,* 1960–1073.

Tarakeshwar, N., Hansen, N., Kochman, A., & Sikkema, K. J. (2005). Gender, ethnicity and spiritual coping among bereaved HIV-positive individuals. *Mental Health, Religion, & Culture, 8,* 109–125.

van der Houwen, K., Stroebe, M., Stroebe, W., Schut, H., van den Bout, J., & Wijngaards-de Meij, L. (2010). Risk factors for bereavement outcome: A multivariate approach. *Death Studies, 34,* 195–220.

Wagner, B., Knaevelsrud, C., & Maercker, A. (2006). Internet-based cognitive-behavioral therapy for complicated grief: A randomized controlled trial. *Death Studies, 30,* 429–453.

Wijngaards-de Meij, L., Stroebe, M., Schut, H., Stroebe, W., van den Bout, J., & Heijden, P. G. M. (2007a). Patterns of attachment and parents' adjustment to the death of their child. *Personality and Social Psychology Bulletin, 33,* 537.

Wijngaards-de Meij, L., Stroebe, M., Schut, H., Stroebe, W., van den Bout, J., & Heijden, P. G. M. (2007b). Neuroticism and attachment insecurity as predictors of bereavement outcome. *Journal of Research and Personality, 41,* 498–505.

Worden, J. W. (2002). *Grief counseling and grief therapy: A handbook for the mental health practitioner* (3rd ed.). New York: Springer Publishing Company.

Wright, A. A., Keating, N. L., Balboni, T. A., Matulonis, U. A., Block, S. D., & Prigerson, H. G. (2010). Place of death: Correlations with quality of life of patients with cancer and predictors of bereaved caregivers' mental health. *Journal of Clinical Oncology, 28,* 1–8. doi: 10.1200/JCO.2009.26.3863.

Wright, A. A., Zhang, B., Alaka, R., Mack, J. W., Trice, E., Balboni, T., . . . Prigerson, H. G. (2008). Associations between end-of-life discussions, patient mental health, medical care near death, and caregiver bereavement adjustment. *JAMA, 300*(14), 1665–1673. doi: 10.1001/jama.300.14.1665.

Index

AANEHS. *See* American Academy of Neurology Ethics and Humanities Subcommittee
ABA. *See* American Bar Association
ACA. *See* American Counseling Association
ACP. *See* advance care planning
activities of daily living (ADL), 8, 145, 187
acupuncture, 113
acute care. *See also* palliative care
   advance care planning, 66
   advance directives in, 65
   DNR orders, 65
   general medicine unit, 66
   medical versus surgical admission, 65
   therapeutic intervention issue, 69–70
acute stress disorder, 107
ADAA. *See* Anxiety Disorders Association of America
addiction, 158, 159
   action, 198
   in chronic pain populations, 157
   at life's end, 197–198
   outcome, 198
   pseudo-addiction, 159
   sexual, 12
ADEC. *See* Association for Death Education and Counseling
ADL. *See* activities of daily living
adolescents. *See also* end of life care
   death system, 123–124
   dying as confluence, 126
   tasks of dying, 124–126
ADVANCE. *See* Advance Directives, Values Assessment, and Communication Enhancement

advance care planning (ACP), 53–54, 189, 193
   completion of advance directives, 58–59
   ethnic differences and disparities, 56–58
   family involvement, 60
   intervention, 66–68
   purpose of, 58
   racial differences, 56–58, 60
advance directives, 53, 160
   in acute care, 65–66
   ADVANCE intervention, 67
   clinicians working in, 65
   coherent verbal interaction, 64
   community-dwelling sample, 56
   completion of, 53
   culture, 57
   DNR, 54, 64
   EOL planning, 56, 63
   ethnic minorities, 56
   full code patients' descriptions, 55
   to health care team, 161
   health literacy, 57
   ICU, 55
   influence of depression, 63
   life-sustaining medical treatments, 56
   in long-term care, 64
   using nonopioid or opioid analgesics, 65
   nursing home residents, 63
   Pc-ACP approach, 67–68
   personal vulnerability, 56
   prevalence rates, 64
   proxy-reported data, 54–55
   PSDA, 67

advance directives (*Contd.*)
    qualitative analysis, 55
    racial and ethnic minorities, 57
    SPIRIT intervention, 68
    SUPPORT intervention, 66
    treatment preference, 58
Advance Directives, Values Assessment, and Communication Enhancement (ADVANCE), 67
aggressive treatments, 29, 30, 31, 35, 128, 129
AIDS dementia complex, 169
ALFs. *See* assisted living facilities
ALS. *See* amyotrophic lateral sclerosis
Alzheimer's disease, 165, 168, 169
AMA Council. *See* American Medical Association Council
American Academy of Neurology Ethics and Humanities Subcommittee (AANEHS), 175
American Bar Association (ABA), 62
American Counseling Association (ACA), 5, 11
American Medical Association Council (AMA Council), 17
American Psychological Association (APA), 101, 143, 166. *See also* Working Group
    Division of Trauma Psychology, 154, 157
    guidelines for psychologists, 62
amyotrophic lateral sclerosis (ALS), 4, 109
antidepressants, 106
anxiety disorders, 145. *See also* mood disorders
    categories, 146
    clinical, 107
    elder care, 145
    reasons, 145, 146
    treatment, 146–147
Anxiety Disorders Association of America (ADAA), 145

APA. *See* American Psychological Association
assessment, 63, 64, 143, 199
    areas of, 45
    clients' concerns, 31
    of depression, 148
    instrument's use, 117–118
    tools, 151, 190–192
assisted living facilities (ALFs), 186
Association for Death Education and Counseling (ADEC), 17, 18, 19
authentic presence, 42

BDI-II. *See* Beck Depression Inventory-II
Beck Depression Inventory-II (BDI-II), 148
bereavement, 205
    associated intervention, 215
    CGT, 218–219
    FFGT, 216–218
    initial grief responses, 213
    intense grief reactions, 214–215
    negative cognitions, 213–214
    reconstruction approaches, 219–224
    risk factors, 212–213
    risk index, 190
    sense making, 214
bio–psycho–socio–spiritual issues, 104, 112. *See also* end-of-life decisions
    comorbid psychological conditions, 105–108
    cultural factors, 111, 112
    fear of loss of control, 110
    financial concerns, 111
    physical pain and suffering, 104, 105
    psychological issues, 108–110
    quality of life, 113
    religious and spiritual belief systems, 109
bipolar disorders, 107, 147, 148
boundary crossings, 17, 18, 21

cardiopulmonary resuscitation (CPR), 4–5, 7, 8, 170

caregivers, 185
  assessment tools, 190–192
  counseling, 185–186
  family, 185
  formal, 187
  informal, 187
  mistake, 133
  needs and distress, 185
  reciprocal suffering, 185
Caregivers' burden scale in end-of-life care (CBS-EOLC), 190
Caregiving, 187, 196
  ALF, 186
  assessment tools, 190–192
  bereavement risk, 189–190
  challenges, 188
  CMS, 187
  communication concerns, 189
  family caregivers, 187
  family members, 187, 188
  illness-related problems, 189
  palliative care, 186–187
  personal hygiene, 188
  primary, 188
  sense of new normalcy, 188
  stressors, 188–189
  transformative aspects, 188
  uncertainties, 187
CBS-EOLC. *See* Caregivers' burden scale in end-of-life care
CBT. *See* cognitive behavioral therapy
CDC. *See* Centers for Disease Control and Prevention
Center for Epidemiological Studies-Depression Scale (CES-D), 148
Centers for Disease Control and Prevention (CDC), 155
Centers for Medicare and Medicaid Services (CMS), 176, 187
CES-D. *See* Center for Epidemiological Studies-Depression Scale
CFRA. *See* checklist of family relational abilities
CG. *See* complicated grief

CGT. *See* complicated grief treatment
checklist of family relational abilities (CFRA), 190
children. *See also* end-of-life care (EOLC)
  death system, 123–124
  dying as confluence, 126
  tasks of dying, 124–126
clarity of termination, 19
client's capacity, 103
  instrument use with dying clients, 117–118
  MacCAT-T instrument, 103
clinical depression, 106, 142, 148
  dignity therapy, 107
  IMCP, 106, 107
  MCGP, 106
  treatment in older adults, 150
clinicians, 4, 54
  diagnostic category, 143–144
  focus on shared decision making, 59
  issues for, 57–58
  role for, 54, 56, 154, 160–161, 206
  working in health care settings, 68
  working with cancer patients, 107
CMS. *See* Centers for Medicare and Medicaid Services
cognitive behavioral therapy (CBT), 219
cognitive impairment, 165, 174
  advocacy, 173, 177, 178–179
  barriers to end-of-life care, 178
  behavioral disturbances, 171
  causes, 165
  CMS Manual System, 177
  counseling interventions, 171
  cultural beliefs, 173, 174
  decision makers, 176
  dementia, 171, 173
  depression, 165, 171
  DHHS, 176
  health care and perceptions, 175
  hospice care for individuals, 177
  individual with, 171
  irreversible, 168–169
  legal/ethical issues, 175–176
  life review, 172

cognitive impairment (*Contd.*)
  long-term approaches, 171
  MAC and LCD, 176
  memory skills, 176
  mental health services, 177
  multidisciplinary treatment team, 178
  national policy level, 178–179
  opportunities, 179
  play therapy, 172
  problem-focused therapy, 172–173
  regulatory issues, 176–177
  reversible and irreversible, 166–168
  spaced retrieval, 172
  terminal clients, 175
  validation therapy, 172
cognitive restructuring technique, 219
comorbid psychological conditions, 105, 106
  clinical depression, 106–107
  mood disorders, 107
  pain medication, 108
  personality disorders, 108
  psychosis, 107, 108
competence, 5
  cultural, 59
  death, 3, 19
complicated grief (CG), 206
  death-related risk factor, 209–212
  features, 206, 207
  predisposing factors, 207–209
  pre-loss risk factor checklist for, 213
  risk factors in bereavement, 212, 213–215
  symptoms, 207
complicated grief treatment (CGT), 218
confidentiality, 14, 19
counseling caregivers, 191
  assessment tools for, 191
  interventions for, 194
counselors. *See also* caregivers
  boundary crossings, 17
  main things for, 106
  at multidisciplinary treatment team, 178
  roles, 32–33, 114, 118

counter-transference issue, 21
CPR. *See* cardiopulmonary resuscitation
Creutzfeldt–Jakob disease, 169
culture, 33–34, 57
  care, 88
  cognitive impairment patients, 173
  death phobic, 122
  ethnic, 36
  generalizations, 10
Cyclothymic Disorder, 147, 148

death competence, 3, 19
death phobic cultures, 122
death proximity, 3
  death competence, 3
  ethical challenges and dilemmas, 3
  hospital based palliative care, 3–4
  outpatient end of life counseling, 4
death system, 122, 123
  children and adolescents, 123–124
  emerging and young adults, 126–128
  middle age and dying, 130–131
  older adults, 132–133
degree of power, 18
delirium, 150, 166
  causes, 150, 151
  characterization, 151
  diagnosis, 151
  treatment, 151, 152
dementia, 152
  and delirium, 152
  and depression, 171
  types, 169
Department of Health and Human Services (DHHS), 176
dependence and guilt at life's end, 195
  action, 196–197
  counseling issues, 196
  outcome, 197
depressive disorders, 106, 147
  diagnosis, 148
despair, 109
developmental-dying task approach, 122

DHHS. *See* Department of Health and Human Services
Diagnostic and Statistical Manual (DSM), 143, 144, 145
Diagnostic and Statistical Manual of Mental Disorders IV (DSM-IV), 143
dignity therapy (DT), 107, 193
direct external coercion, 116, 117. *See also* indirect external coercion
DNR/CC. *See* Do Not Resucitate/Comfort Care
DNR order. *See* do not resuscitate order (DNR order)
Do Not Resucitate/Comfort Care (DNR/CC), 170
do not resuscitate order (DNR order), 8, 53, 54, 160
DSM-IV. *See Diagnostic and Statistical Manual of Mental Disorders IV*
DSM nosology, 145, 147, 153
   depressive disorders, 147
   ego-dystonic impairment of functioning, 145
   personality disorder types, 153
DT. *See* dignity therapy
dying as confluence, 123
   children and adolescents, 126
   emerging and young adults, 129–130
   middle age and dying, 131, 132
   older adults, 135
dysthymia, 107

elder care, 145
elder law clinic geropsychology consultation, 61
   ABA and APA, 62
   decision-making capacity, 61
   decisional capacity, 61
   undue influence, 62, 63
emerging adults, 127. *See also* adolescents
   death system, 126, 127, 128
   dying as confluence, 129–130
   tasks of dying, 128–129

emotional memory work, 218
end of life (EOL), 206
   decision making, 6, 210–211
   ethics, 210
   medical care, 210
   principles of family therapy, 217
end-of-life care (EOLC), 25, 121, 186
   age-related tasks, 122
   case study, 43–44
   death system, 122, 123
   developmental tasks, 123
   dying as confluence, 123
   ethics, 210
   family involvement, 60
   goals, 25
   medical care, 210
   mental health symptom management, 141
   racial and/or ethnic influence, 35–37
   racial/ethnic and cultural diversity, 32–33
   racial/ethnic disparities, 34–35
   tasks of dying, 122, 123
end-of-life decision making, 101, 210, 211
   bio–psycho–socio–spiritual issues, 104–113
   client's capacity, 103, 104
   preliminary considerations, 102
   social support system issues, 113–116
   systemic and environmental issues, 116–117
end-of-life experiences. *See also* spiritual and religious diversity
   culture, 33–34
   ethnicity, 33
   race, 33
   racial and ethnic disparities, 34–35
   racial and/or ethnic influence, 35–37
   special considerations, 38
   understanding, 33
end-of-life trajectories, 27–28
   life-threatening conditions, 27, 29
   medical conditions effect, 29

end-of-life trajectories (*Contd.*)
   palliative care, 29
   transitions between care settings, 29–30
energy therapy, 113
EOL. *See* end-of-life
EOLC. *See* end-of-life care
estrangement, 14
   action, 198
   at life's end, 197
   outcome, 198
ethnicity, 33
   bereavement complication, 208–209
   cultural factors, 111
   differences in ACP, 57
exposure, 219

family-focused grief therapy (FFGT), 193, 216
   challenges, 216, 217
   classification, 216
   therapeutic processes, 216, 217, 218
family–provider conferences, 193
family relationships index (FRI), 216
fear of loss of control, 110
FFGT. *See* family-focused grief therapy
fidelity, 16–17
Five P Model, 11, 13
   person, 14
   place, 15
   principles, 16–19
   problem, 14–16
   process, 19–22
frailty group, 27, 28
FRI. *See* family relationships index
Frontotemporal dementia, 169

geriatrics clinic client with mental illness, 63–64
grieving, 109–110, 172, 206, 216, 219
groups, 81
   forming, 81, 82
   norming, 82
   performing, 83
   storming, 82

HCP. *See* health care provider (HCP)
health care institutions, 53
health care provider (HCP), 53, 68
   hands-on-care, 185
   involvement, 59
   woman's advance directive, 70
health care teams, 76, 77. *See also* team organization
   affecting factors, 81–83
   attitudes about palliative care, 88–90
   complexity, 90
   conflict management, 91, 92, 93
   counseling patients, 85–87
   emphasis on psychopathology, 85
   enhancing methods, 90–91
   good working relationships, 94
   health care settings, 83–90
   interdisciplinary teams, 77, 78
   interprofessional training programs, 88
   multidisciplinary teams, 77
   organization, 80, 81
   organizational policies, 83, 84
   providing palliative care, 78–79
   relationship building, 94
   social workers report, 85
   tension, 88
   training models, 84
   transdisciplinary teams, 78
hopelessness, 31, 109
hospice, 29, 79
hospital based palliative care, 3, 4. *See also* palliative care
   ADL, 8
   EOL medical decision making, 6
   interdisciplinary approach, 4
   need for counseling, 11
   need for extensive counseling, 11
   patient's self-determination, 4, 5, 6
   research, 10
   self determination protection, 6–7
   treatment futile, 9
Huntington's disease, 169
hypnosis, 113

IADL. *See* instrumental activities of daily living
IASP. *See* International Association for the Study of Pain
ICU. *See* intensive care unit
IDM. *See* informed decision making
imaginal revisiting, 218
IMCP. *See* individualized version of MCGP
indirect external coercion, 116
individualized version of MCGP (IMCP), 106
informed decision making (IDM), 59
instrumental activities of daily living (IADL), 187
intensive care unit (ICU), 55, 186
interdisciplinary teams, 77, 78
International Association for the Study of Pain (IASP), 141
interpersonal psychotherapy (IPT), 219
interventions
 ACP, 193
 ADVANCE, 67
 for counseling caregivers, 194–195
 DT, 193
 family–provider conferences, 193
 FFGT, 193
 legacy, 195
 listening to silence, 192
 LWHP, 193
 nonabandonment, 192
 psychoeducation, 192–193
 QPS, 193
 reminiscence therapy, 195
 SPIRIT, 68
 structured, 192
 SUPPORT, 66
 therapeutic, 69
intubation. *See* cardiopulmonary resuscitation
invasive mechanical ventilation. *See* cardiopulmonary resuscitation (CPR)
IPT. *See* interpersonal psychotherapy

irreversible cognitive impairment, 166, 168. *See also* reversible cognitive impairment
 causes, 169
 dementia and depression, 171
 memory impairment, 169
 prognosis and progression, 169
 symptoms, 169

kinship, 208

LCD. *See* local coverage determination
Lewy body dementia, 169
life review, 41, 134, 172
lifespan considerations, 136–138
 children and adolescents, 123–126
 emerging and young adults, 126–130
 middle age people, 130–132
 older adults, 132–135
living with hope program (LWHP), 193, 194
local coverage determination (LCD), 176
long-term care (LTC), 170
loss of autonomy. *See* fear of loss of control
loss of dignity. *See* fear of loss of control
Lou Gehrig's disease. *See* amyotrophic lateral sclerosis (ALS)
LTC. *See* long-term care (LTC)
LWHP. *See* living with hope program

MAC. *See* Medicare Administrative Contractor
MacArthur Competence Assessment Tool–Treatment (MacCAT-T), 103–104
manic-depression. *See* bipolar disorders
Marwit Meuser caregiver grief inventory (MMCGI), 190, 191
MCGP. *See* Meaning-Centered Group Psychotherapy
Meaning-Centered Group Psychotherapy (MCGP), 106, 109
medical power of attorney (MPOA), 7

Medicare Administrative Contractor (MAC), 176
Memorial Delirium Assessment Scale, 151
mental health
  claims submission, 176
  depression, 62
  needs, 143
  practitioner's work, 148
  providers, 75, 83, 92
  severe mental illness, 63
  symptom presentation, 143
  veterans with schizophrenia, 63
Mental Health America (MHA), 148
mental health management, 141, 142
  advance directives, 160, 161
  anxiety disorders, 145–147
  decision making, 143
  delirium, 150–152
  diagnosis, 143–145
  mental health needs, 143
  mood disorders, 147–150
  personality disorders, 152–154
  substance dependence, 157–160
  trauma, 154–157
MHA. *See* Mental Health America
middle age and dying. *See also* emerging adults
  death system, 130–131
  dying as confluence, 131, 132
  generativity versus stagnation, 130
  tasks of dying, 131, 132
MMCGI. *See* Marwit Meuser caregiver grief inventory
mood disorders, 107–108, 147
  bipolar disorders, 147
  cyclothymic disorder, 147, 148
  depressive disorders, 147
  diagnosis, 148–149
  treatment, 149–150
motor vehicle accidents (MVA), 208
MPOA. *See* medical power of attorney
multidisciplinary teams, 77
multiple relationships, 17, 18
MVA. *See* motor vehicle accidents

National Institute of Mental Health (NIMH), 147
neuroticism, 153
NIMH. *See* National Institute of Mental Health
nonabandonment, 192
normal anxiety, 146

older adults. *See also* end-of-life care (EOLC); middle age and dying
  death system, 132–133
  dying as confluence, 135
  end-of-life trajectories, 27–30
  family concerns, 31–32
  physical concerns, 30–31
  psychological concerns, 31
  special needs, 26–28
  spiritual concerns, 31, 32
  tasks of dying, 133–134
organ failure group, 27, 28
outpatient end of life counseling, 4, 11. *See also* palliative care
  Five P Model, 13–22
  prostate cancer, 11, 12, 13

pain medication, 108
palliative care, 4, 29, 186–187. *See* health care teams
  end-of-life care, 79
  hospice services, 79
  primary treatment team, 78
  in serious illness and dying stages, 79
pancytopenia, 8
Parkinson's disease, 165, 169, 197
patient-centered advance care planning approach (Pc-ACP approach), 67–68
patient dignity inventory, 190, 192
patient's capacity, 5. *See also* client's capacity
  assessments, 6
  components, 5
  decisional capacity, 61
  evaluations, 61–64
  LCDs use, 176

Patient Self Determination Act
    (PSDA), 53
  requirements, 53
  SUPPORT Principal Investigators, 66
patient's self-determination, 4, 5
  capacity, 5, 6
  competence, 5
  protection, 6, 7
Pc-ACP approach. *See* patient-centered
    advance care planning approach
pediatric hospice, 124
personal hygiene, 188
personality disorders, 108, 152. *See also*
    mood disorders
  diagnosis, 152–153
  treatment, 153–154
  types, 153
PGD. *See* prolonged grief disorder
Physician Orders for Life-Sustaining
    Treatment (POLST), 7
play therapy, 172
POLST. *See* Physician Orders for
    Life-Sustaining Treatment
postmortem disclosures, 17, 18
posttraumatic stress disorder (PTSD),
    107, 154
predisposing risk factors, 207. *See also*
    complicated grief (CG)
  attachment styles, 209
  gender differences, 207–208
  kinship, 208
  racial and ethnicity, 208–209
present awareness, 42
previous anxiety, 146
Primary Care Evaluation of Mental
    Disorders (PRIME-MD), 148–149
problem-focused therapy, 172–173
prolonged grief disorder (PGD), 206
provider–client relationship, 14, 15
  in end-of-life counseling, 16
  pysical contact, 15
provider–client relationship, 14–15, 16
PSDA. *See* Patient Self Determination Act
pseudo-addiction, 159
psychosis, 107, 108

psychotherapy, 3, 177
PTSD. *See* posttraumatic stress disorder

question prompt sheet (QPS),
    193, 194

race, 33
  cultural diversity, 32–33
  differences in ACP, 57
  generalizations, 10
  susceptibility to bereavement
      complication, 208–209
reactive anxiety, 146
religiosity, 26, 31, 39, 40
reminiscence therapy, 195
reversible cognitive impairment, 166
  causes, 167
  contributing factors, 166
  delirium, 166
  multidisciplinary team approach, 168
  rapid-onset of, 166
role release, 78

shared decision making. *See also* advance
    directives
  Caucasian dyads, 60
  EOL decision making, 60
  IDM, 59
  physician/HCP involvement, 59
  preventive health behavior, 58
  USPSTF, 59
  Wisconsin longitudinal study, 58

Sharing Patients' Illness Representations
    to Increase Trust (SPIRIT), 68
situational revisiting, 218
skilled nursing facility (SNF), 167
SNF. *See* skilled nursing facility
social death, 122, 133
social support system issues, 113
  consideration of significant others,
      113, 114
  interviews with significant others, 116
  involvement of significant others,
      114, 115

Social work assessment tool (SWAT), 190, 191
solution-focused approach, 156
spaced retrieval technique (SR technique), 172
SPIRIT. *See* Sharing Patients' Illness Representations to Increase Trust
spiritual and religious diversity, 37, 39
   practice recommendations, 41–42
   religion and spirituality roles, 40–41
   religiosity, 39
   spiritual care interventions, 41
   spirituality, 39
   spiritual pain, 39–40
SR technique. *See* spaced retrieval technique
stressors, 94, 188–189
Study to Understand Prognoses and Preferences for Outcomes and Risks of Treatment (SUPPORT), 66
substance abuse and dependence, 157, 158
   diagnosis, 158, 159
   substance abuser, 160
   treatment, 159–160
substance abuser, 160
sudden death, 27, 28
SUPPORT. *See* Study to Understand Prognoses and Preferences for Outcomes and Risks of Treatment
SWAT. *See* Social work assessment tool
symptomatic anxiety, 146

tasks of dying, 122, 123
   children and adolescents, 124–126
   emerging and young adults, 128–129
   middle age and dying, 131, 132
   older adults, 133–134
team organization, 80–81
   forming, 81, 82
   norming, 82
   performing, 83
   productivity, 81
   storming, 82
   team development, 81
terminal illness, 27, 28, 161, 187
   dysthymia, 107
   hospice services, 29
   mental health providers, 75
   pain, 157
transdisciplinary teams, 78
trauma, 154
   diagnosis, 155–156
   impact of trauma affects, 155
   treatment, 156, 157

unit of care, 22
U. S. Preventive Services Task Force (USPSTF), 59
USPSTF. *See* U. S. Preventive Services Task Force

validation therapy, 172
Vascular dementia, 169
violent death loss, 211

World Health Organization (WHO), 29, 187
Working Group, 101
   bio–psycho–socio–spiritual issues, 104–113
   categories in, 102
   social support system issues, 113–116
   systemic and environmental issues, 116–117

young adults. *See also* children and adolescents
   CG in, 208
   death system, 127, 128
   dying as confluence, 129–130
   tasks of dying, 128–129

www.ingramcontent.com/pod-product-compliance
Ingram Content Group UK Ltd.
Pitfield, Milton Keynes, MK11 3LW, UK
UKHW021833140426
5217IPUK00021B/1424